MUSCLE &FITNESS
hers
101 GET-LEAN
WORKOUTS AND STRATEGIES

ACKNOWLEDGMENTS

This publication is based on articles written by **Michael Berg; Jordana Brown; Mike Carlson; Ian Cohen; Karla Dial; Allan Donnelly; Kathleen Ferguson; Rob Fitzgerald; Dana Leone; Andrea Platzman, M.S., R.D.; Sommer Robertson; Jim Stoppani; Andrew Vontz;** and **Joe Wuebben**

Cover photography by **Chris Fortuna**

Photography and illustrations by: **James + Therese, Art Brewer, Michael Darter, Ian Logan, Jim Purdum, Marc Royce, Erica Schultz,** and **Pavel Ythjall**

Project editor is **Joe Wuebben**

Project creative director is **Anthony Scerri**

Project copy editor is **Cat Perry**

Project photo assistant is **Amy Wolff**

Founding chairman is **Joe Weider.** Chairman and CEO of American Media, Inc., is **David Pecker.**

This book is available in quantity at special discounts for your group or organization. For further information, contact:

Triumph Books
814 North Franklin Street
Chicago, IL 60610
(312) 337-0747
www.triumphbooks.com

ISBN: 978-1-60078-737-9

Printed in USA.

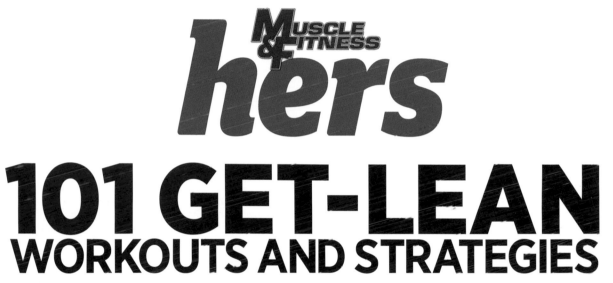

101 GET-LEAN
WORKOUTS AND STRATEGIES

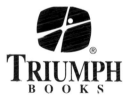

TRIUMPH
BOOKS

TRIUMPHBOOKS**.COM**

Contents

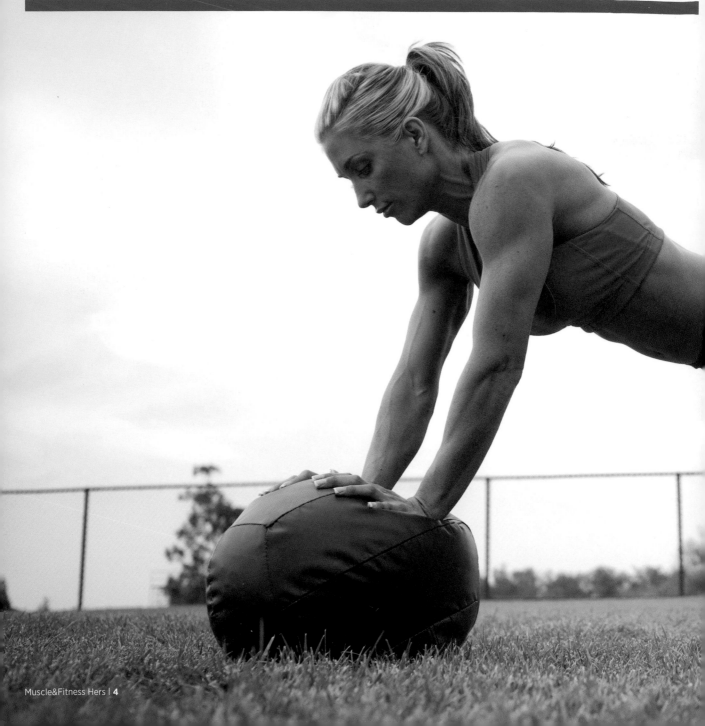

Four Weeks to Fit!

Get your body back with this training, nutrition, and supplement plan designed to help you lose weight and build muscle—fast!

You did it again, didn't you? You've overindulged recently on big lunches and dinners, decadent desserts, and maybe a few too many cocktails. Then, suddenly, one day you woke up with an extra 10 pounds staring back at you in the mirror. So you made a decision to trade your debauchery for the StepMill and clean eating—*again*—knowing it may take months to get back to where you were. But what if you don't want to wait that long? That's where we come in. With the help of trainer and nutritionist Kim Oddo, who has worked with some of the world's top figure and bikini competitors, we'll show you how to get your body back in only four weeks with this comprehensive crash-course training and nutrition program. Yes, it'll have your body sweating and (at times) your stomach grumbling, but in 28 days you'll be back to where you were before you got off track—if not better.

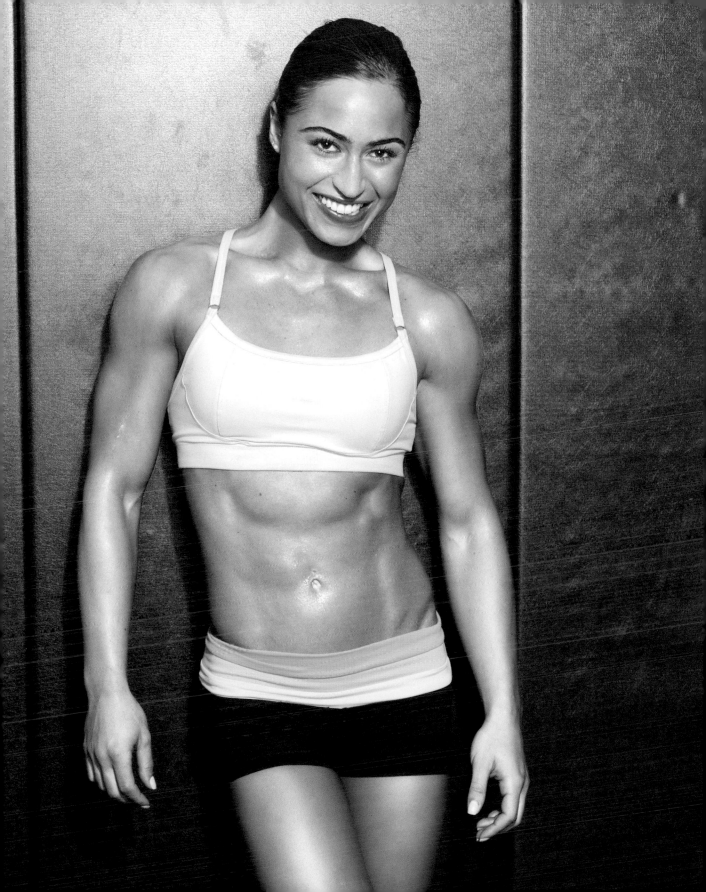

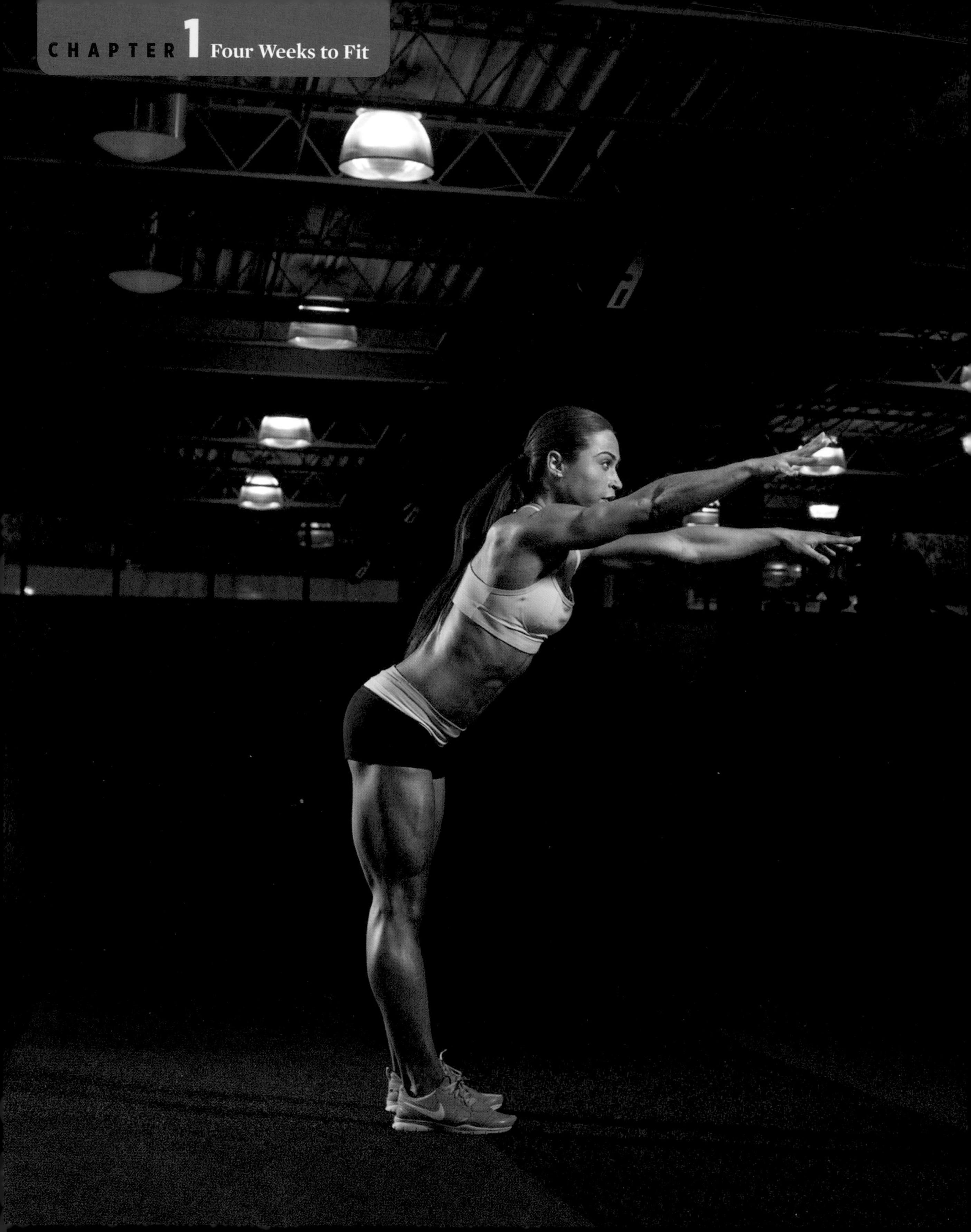

THE
Workout
Split

WEEKS 1-2
DAY 1
Upper-body Circuit, Abs
DAY 2
Lower-body Circuit
DAY 3
Cardio, Abs
DAY 4
Upper-body Circuit, Abs
DAY 5
Lower-body Circuit
DAY 6
Cardio, Abs
DAY 7
Rest

WEEKS 3-4
DAY 1
Upper-body Circuit, Abs
DAY 2
Lower-body Plyometrics
DAY 3
Cardio, Abs
DAY 4
Upper-body Plyometrics, Abs
DAY 5
Lower-body Circuit
DAY 6
Cardio, Abs
DAY 7
Rest

OVERHEAD MEDICINE BALL THROW

• Stand 8-10 feet in front of a concrete wall with feet slightly wider than shoulder width.

• Hold a medicine ball with your palms facing, and lift it above your head with arms extended.

• Bend your knees slightly as you lean back until you feel a slight stretch in your abs.

• Flex forward and throw the ball as hard as possible against the wall.

• Catch the ball on the return and repeat for reps.

Four Weeks to Fit Program

WEEKS 1–2

> Use light weight and higher reps at the beginning of the workout to help enhance blood flow to muscles and burn more calories as you train.

> With each circuit you'll go heavier and use lower reps to stimulate your fast-twitch muscle fibers and keep your body in fat-burning mode after the workout is over.

> Focus on compound movements to maximize the amount of work done in this short, full-body routine.

> To keep your heart rate up, you'll perform five minutes of cardio between each circuit at 70–75% of your maximum heart rate (MHR).

> Use an average tempo like 2:1:2 (two seconds to lower the weight, one second pause, and two seconds to lift it) to ensure you perform each exercise properly.

> Perform 45–60 minutes of cardio on your cardio days (Days 3 and 6), working at 75% of your MHR.

Upper-Body Circuit (Day 1)

EXERCISE	Circuit 1* REPS	Circuit 2* REPS	Circuit 3* REPS	Circuit 4* REPS
Barbell Bentover Row	12	10	8	8
Seated Cable Row	12	10	8	8
Barbell Bench Press	12	10	8	8
Seated Overhead	12	10	8	8
Barbell Press	12	10	8	8
Dumbbell Lateral Raise	12	10	8	8
Triceps Pressdown	12	10	8	8
Barbell Curl	12	10	8	8

*Between each circuit, complete five minutes on treadmill, StepMill, or elliptical at 70–75% MHR.

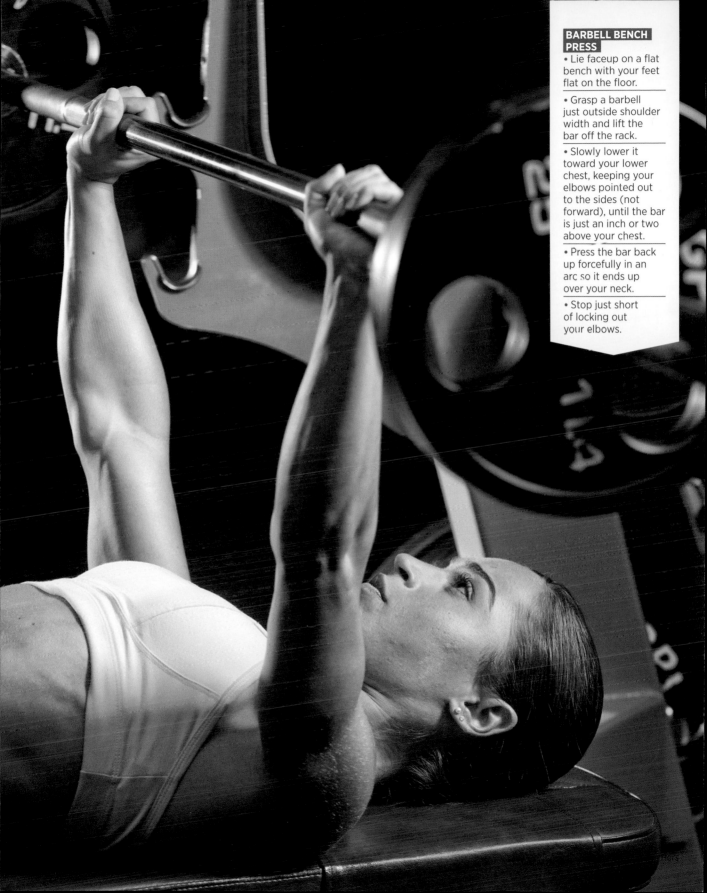

BARBELL BENCH PRESS

- Lie faceup on a flat bench with your feet flat on the floor.

- Grasp a barbell just outside shoulder width and lift the bar off the rack.

- Slowly lower it toward your lower chest, keeping your elbows pointed out to the sides (not forward), until the bar is just an inch or two above your chest.

- Press the bar back up forcefully in an arc so it ends up over your neck.

- Stop just short of locking out your elbows.

STIFF-LEG DEADLIFT

• Stand erect holding a barbell with a shoulder-width, overhand grip, and feet six to eight inches apart.

• Keeping your chest high, abs tight, and knees slightly bent, lean forward at the hips, letting the bar naturally track away from your body.

• Pause when you feel a good stretch, then carefully reverse the motion by contracting your glutes and hamstrings, allowing the bar to come closer to your body as you approach the top position.

• Squeeze your abs, back, and glutes at the top.

FOUR WEEKS TO FIT DIET

As with the training portion of this program, the diet is broken down into two phases over four weeks.

PHASE 1: WEEKS 1–2

> You must eat fewer calories than your body is used to in order to drop body fat. When a calorie deficit is created, the body responds by collecting from fat reserves, and you get leaner. In this phase, you'll eat between 1,400 and 1,500 calories per day.

> You'll consume ample amounts of protein—the building block of muscle—to ensure you're burning off body fat while sparing muscle. This will be coupled with keeping your carbs and fat intake to moderate levels.

MONDAY
Breakfast
1 tsp cinnamon
3 egg whites, scrambled or boiled
⅓ cup oatmeal, quick, measured uncooked
Late-morning Snack
1 tbsp peanut butter, natural
2 rice cakes, brown rice or multigrain
1 scoop whey protein

Lunch
2 tbsp balsamic vinegar
½ cup brown rice, cooked
4 oz shrimp
1 small salad, with tomato and onion
Midday Snack
4 oz ground turkey breast, 99% fat-free
4 oz sweet potato, baked and skinless

Dinner
10 almonds
4 oz asparagus
4 oz halibut
Nighttime Snack
1 tbsp peanut butter, natural
1 scoop whey protein
¼ cup plain, low-fat yogurt
TOTALS: 1,442 Calories, 158g Protein, 114g Carbs, 35g Fat

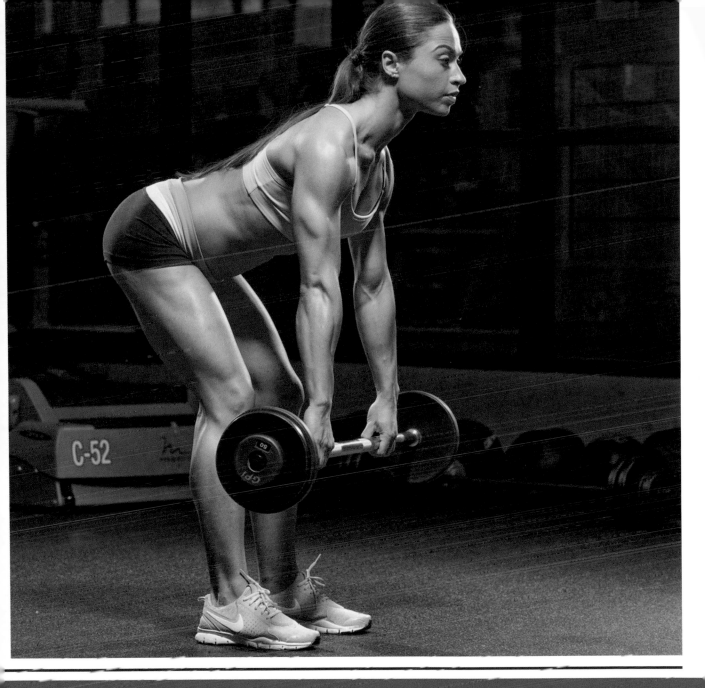

TUESDAY
Breakfast
3 egg whites, scrambled or boiled
1½ oz Cream of Rice, measured uncooked
Late-morning Snack
1 tbsp almond butter, natural
2 rice cakes, brown rice or multigrain
1 scoop whey protein

Lunch
1 soft corn tortilla, 7-inch diameter
4 oz chicken breast, white meat
½ cup zucchini
Midday Snack
4 oz ground turkey breast, 99% fat-free
4 oz sweet potato, baked skinless
Dinner
10 almonds

6 oz broccoli
4 oz halibut
Nighttime Snack
1 oz avocado
1 scoop whey protein
¼ cup plain, low-fat yogurt
TOTALS: 1,433 Calories, 164g Protein, 121g Carbs, 34g Fat

WEDNESDAY
Breakfast
3 egg whites, scrambled

or boiled
¼ cup grits, quick, measured uncooked
Late-morning Snack
1 tbsp peanut butter, natural
2 rice cakes, brown rice or multigrain
1 scoop whey protein
Lunch
2 tbsp balsamic vinegar
½ cup brown rice, cooked

4 oz chicken breast, white meat
1½ cups baby spinach
Midday Snack
4 oz ground turkey breast, 99% fat-free
4 oz sweet potato, baked skinless
Dinner
2 tbsp balsamic vinegar
10 almonds
1 medium salad, with tomato and onion

4 oz shrimp
Nighttime Snack
1 tbsp peanut butter, natural
1 scoop whey protein
¼ cup plain, low-fat yogurt
TOTALS: 1,408 Calories, 164g Protein, 144g Carbs, 34g Fat

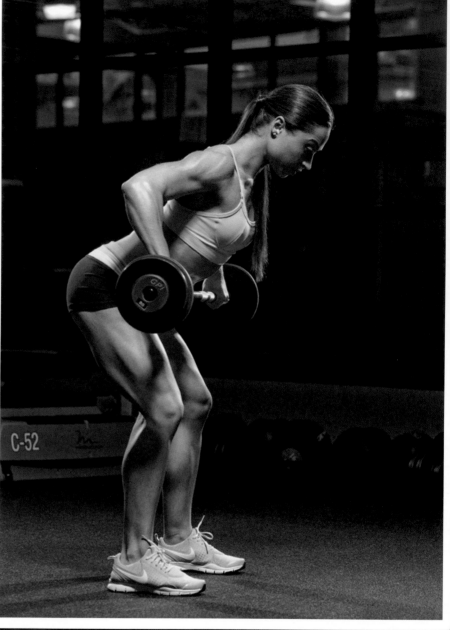

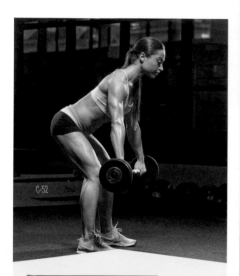

BARBELL BENTOVER ROW

• Stand holding a barbell with your feet shoulder-width apart and bend forward at about a 45-degree angle.

• Keeping your back stable and head up, pull the bar toward your body until it touches your belly button.

• Squeeze your shoulder blades together and pause for a moment at the top of the movement.

• Slowly return to the start position, making sure to stretch your lats fully at the bottom.

THURSDAY
Breakfast
1 tsp cinnamon
3 egg whites, scrambled or boiled
⅓ cup oatmeal, quick, measured uncooked
Late-morning Snack
1 tbsp peanut butter, natural
2 rice cakes, brown rice or multigrain
1 scoop whey protein

Lunch
4 oz sweet potato, baked and skinless
4 oz chicken breast, white meat
4 oz asparagus
Midday Snack
4 oz turkey breast, white meat
½ cup brown rice
Dinner
2 tbsp balsamic vinegar
10 almonds

1 medium salad, with tomato and onion
5 oz tilapia
Nighttime Snack
1 tbsp almond butter, natural
1 scoop whey protein
¼ cup plain, low-fat yogurt
TOTALS: 1,491 Calories, 198g Protein, 94g Carbs, 35g Fat

FRIDAY
Breakfast
1 tsp cinnamon
3 egg whites, scrambled or boiled
½ cup oat bran
Late-morning Snack
1 tbsp almond butter, natural
2 rice cakes, brown rice or multigrain
1 scoop whey protein

Lunch
½ cup brown rice, cooked
4 oz chicken breast, white meat
4 oz green beans
Midday Snack
4 oz ground turkey breast, 99% fat-free
4 oz sweet potato, baked and skinless
Dinner
1 oz avocado

4 oz asparagus
4 oz halibut
Nighttime Snack
1 tbsp peanut butter, natural
1 scoop whey protein
¼ cup plain, low-fat yogurt
TOTALS: 1,474 Calories, 172g Protein, 123g Carbs, 38g Fat

Lower-Body Circuit (Day 2)

EXERCISE	Circuit 1* REPS	Circuit 2* REPS	Circuit 3* REPS	Circuit 4* Reps
Leg Press	12	10	8	8
Leg Extension	12	10	8	8
Lying Leg Curl	12	10	8	8
Stiff-leg Deadlift	12	10	8	8
Standing Calf Raise	12	10	8	8

Between each circuit, complete five minutes on treadmill, StepMill, or elliptical at 70–75% MHR.

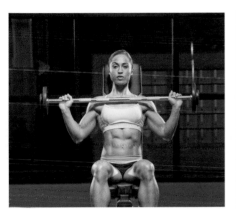
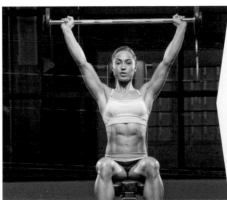

SEATED OVERHEAD BARBELL PRESS
• Sit on a bench that adjusts to 90 degrees.

• Take an overhand grip slightly wider than shoulder width and start with the bar under your chin and just above your upper chest.

• Press the bar straight up overhead until your arms are fully extended but not completely locked out.

• Slowly lower the bar back to the start position and repeat.

LEG PRESS
• Sit squarely in a leg-press machine and place your feet on the platform, shoulder-width apart.

• Keeping your chest up and your lower back slightly arched, lift the sled, and unlatch the safeties.

• Bend your knees to lower the weight toward you, stopping before your lower back and glutes lift off the pad.

• Pause for a moment, then extend your legs to press the weight up, stopping just short of locking out your knees.

• Squeeze your thighs hard at the top and repeat.

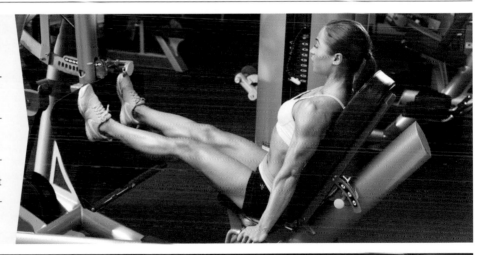

SATURDAY
Breakfast
3 egg whites, scrambled or boiled
2 oz hash browns, home-prepared
Late-morning Snack
1 tbsp peanut butter, natural
2 rice cakes, brown rice or multigrain
1 scoop whey protein

Lunch
2 tbsp balsamic vinegar
½ cup brown rice, cooked
5 oz tilapia
1½ cups baby spinach
Midday Snack
4 oz turkey breast, white meat
4 oz sweet potato, baked and skinless
Dinner
10 almonds

1 cup zucchini
4 oz ground turkey breast, 99% fat-free
Nighttime Snack
1 tbsp almond butter, natural
1 scoop whey protein
¼ cup plain, low-fat yogurt
TOTALS: 1,489 Calories, 175g Protein, 110g Carbs, 41g Fat

SUNDAY
Breakfast
3 egg whites, scrambled or boiled
¼ cup grits, quick, measured uncooked
Late-morning Snack
1 tbsp almond butter, natural
2 rice cakes, brown rice or multigrain
1 scoop whey protein

Lunch
½ cup black beans, boiled
4 oz chicken breast, white meat
4 oz broccoli
Midday Snack
4 oz ground turkey breast, 99% fat-free
½ cup brown rice, cooked
Dinner
2 tbsp balsamic vinegar
10 almonds

1 medium salad, with tomato and onion
4 oz shrimp

Nighttime Snack
1 oz avocado
1 scoop whey protein
¼ cup plain, low-fat yogurt
TOTALS: 1,456 Calories, 168g Protein, 141g Carbs, 33g Fat

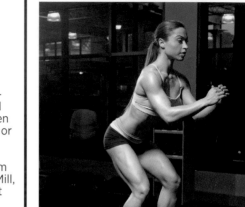

Four Weeks to Fit Program

WEEKS 3-4 // OVERVIEW

> Increase the amount of weight for both your upper- and lower-body circuits (Days 1 and 5, respectively, during weeks 3–4), and go heavier and use lower reps with each circuit.

> After your body has acclimatized to faster-paced workouts, you'll start plyometrics—exercises that are quick, powerful movements that help the muscles store energy for more explosive training.

> Plyos give you a total cardio workout, so you won't have to hit the treadmill afterward unless you feel you need to.

> To keep your heart rate up and calories burning during the workout, you'll perform five minutes of cardio between each circuit on the treadmill, StepMill, or elliptical at 70–75% of your MHR.

> Make sure to warm up for a minimum of five minutes on the treadmill, StepMill, or elliptical before beginning your first circuit.

> Perform 45–60 minutes of cardio on a treadmill, StepMill, or elliptical on your cardio days (days 3 and 6) at 75% of your MHR.

Lower-Body Plyometrics Workout (Day 2)

EXERCISE	Circuit 1* REPS	Circuit 2* REPS	Circuit 3* REPS	Circuit 4* Reps
Box Jump	20	20	15	15
Bench Step-up	20	20	15	15
One-leg Bench Squat	20	20	15	15
Exercise Ball Hip Lift	20	20	15	15
Calf Jump (with/without rope)	30	30	25	25

Between each circuit, complete five minutes on treadmill, StepMill, or elliptical at 70–75% MHR.

BOX JUMP
• Stand in front of a box or aerobics step.

• Sit back into squat position, arms at your sides.

• Straighten your legs and jump up onto the top of the box or step, landing softly and evenly on both feet.

• Jump back down and repeat.

PHASE 2: WEEKS 3-4

> Like Weeks 1–2, Weeks 3–4 are structured to help you lose weight while curtailing losses in lean muscle.
> In this phase, you'll eat between 1,400-1,500 calories per day, as before; however, your macronutrient intake will change.
> Because high-intensity training tears down muscle fibers at a rapid rate, you'll consume a combination of higher protein and healthy fats.
> Carb intake is low to help keep your metabolism humming along. Carbs are still consumed early in the day, but they taper off as insulin sensitivity increases.

MONDAY
Breakfast
3 egg whites, scrambled or boiled
1 tbsp flaxseeds
⅓ cup oatmeal, quick, measured uncooked
Late-morning Snack
3 oz chicken breast, white meat
¾ oz English walnuts, halves

Lunch
1 cup cabbage, raw, shredded
4 oz chicken breast, white meat
2 soft corn tortillas, 7-inch diameter
Midday Snack
½ medium banana
1 tbsp flaxseeds
1½ scoops whey protein

Dinner
2 oz avocado
1 tbsp balsamic vinegar
1 medium salad, with tomato and onion
4 oz turkey breast, white meat
Nighttime Snack
1 tbsp flaxseeds
1½ scoops whey protein
TOTALS: 1,490 Calories, 180g Protein, 90g Carbs, 47g Fat

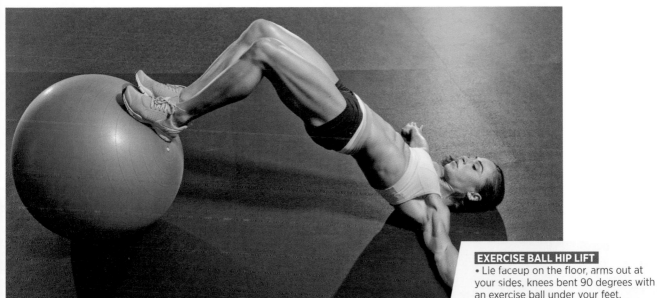

EXERCISE BALL HIP LIFT

• Lie faceup on the floor, arms out at your sides, knees bent 90 degrees with an exercise ball under your feet.

• Dig into the ball with your heels to lift your hips as high as possible.

• Pause for a moment, then lower to just before your glutes touch the floor and repeat.

TUESDAY
Breakfast
3 egg whites, scrambled or boiled
1 tbsp flaxseeds
¼ cup grits, quick, measured uncooked
Late-morning Snack
3 oz chicken breast, white meat
15 almonds

Lunch
1 cup cabbage, raw, shredded
4 oz ground turkey breast, 99% fat-free
2 soft corn tortillas, 7-inch diameter
Midday Snack
3 oz blueberries
1 tbsp flaxseeds
1½ scoops whey protein

Dinner
¾ oz English walnuts, halves
4 oz broccoli
4 oz turkey breast, white meat
Nighttime Snack
1 tbsp peanut butter, natural
1½ scoops whey protein
TOTALS: 1,439 Calories, 179g Protein, 94g Carbs, 50g Fat

WEDNESDAY
Breakfast
3 egg whites, scrambled or boiled
1 tbsp flaxseeds
2 oz hash browns, home-prepared
Late-morning Snack
3 oz chicken breast, white meat
¾ oz English walnuts, halves

Lunch
½ cup zucchini
4 oz turkey breast, white meat
4 oz sweet potato, baked, skinless
Midday Snack
½ medium apple
1 tbsp flaxseeds
1½ scoops whey protein
Dinner
1 oz avocado

4 oz broccoli
3 egg whites, scrambled or boiled
Nighttime Snack
1 tbsp almond butter, natural
1½ scoops whey protein
TOTALS: 1,413 Calories, 160g Protein, 93g Carbs, 52g Fat

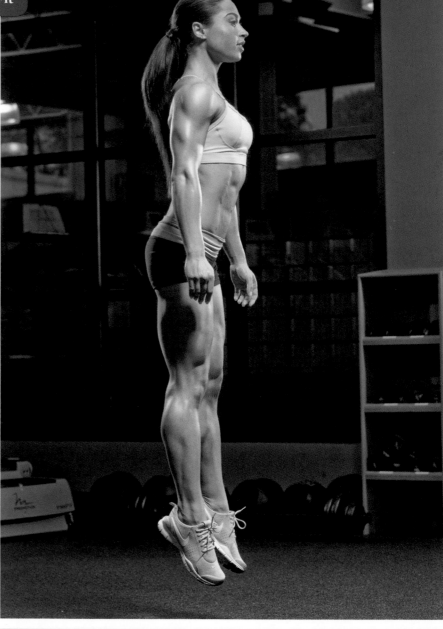

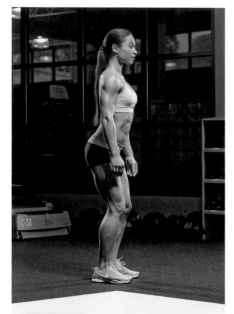

CALF JUMP

• Stand with your feet close together and bend your knees only slightly (this is not meant to be a squatting movement).

• Push through your calves and jump straight up, keeping your upper arms close to your sides.

• Continue making small jumps repeatedly (about three inches high).

THURSDAY
Breakfast
3 egg whites, scrambled or boiled
1 tbsp flaxseeds
⅓ cup oatmeal, quick, measured uncooked
Late-morning Snack
3 oz chicken breast, white meat
2 oz avocado

Lunch
1 cup cabbage, raw, shredded
4 oz chicken breast, white meat
½ cup brown rice, cooked
Midday Snack
½ medium grapefruit
1 tbsp flaxseeds
1½ scoops whey protein

Dinner
¾ oz English walnuts, halves
1 tbsp balsamic vinegar
1½ cups baby spinach
4 oz shrimp
Nighttime Snack
1 tbsp flaxseeds
1½ scoops whey protein
TOTALS: 1,448 Calories, 171g Protein, 82g Carbs, 51g Fat

FRIDAY
Breakfast
3 egg whites, scrambled or boiled
1 tbsp flaxseeds
1.5 oz Cream of Rice, uncooked
Late-morning Snack
4 oz ground turkey breast, 99% fat-free
¾ oz English walnuts, halves

Lunch
4 oz asparagus
4 oz shrimp
4 oz sweet potato, baked and skinless
Midday Snack
½ large orange
1 tbsp peanut butter, natural
1½ scoops whey protein
Dinner
1 oz avocado

4 oz asparagus
5 oz tilapia
Nighttime Snack
1 tbsp flaxseeds
1½ scoops whey protein
TOTALS: 1,480 Calories, 178g Protein, 97g Carbs, 46g Fat

ONE-LEG BENCH SQUAT

• Stand two to three feet in front of a bench with a barbell resting across your upper back and feet shoulder-width apart, toes pointed forward.

• Extend your left leg back, placing the top of your foot on the bench while keeping your right foot firmly planted on the floor.

• With your back flat, squat down until your right thigh is parallel to the floor.

• Press up through your heel, shifting your hips forward and squeezing your glutes to return to standing.

• Switch legs and repeat.

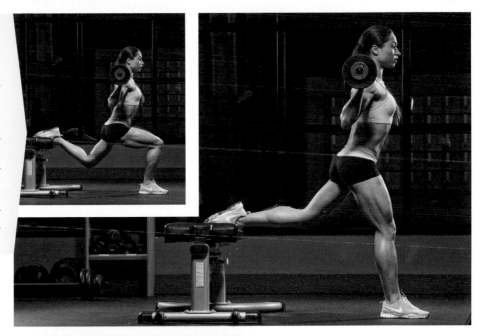

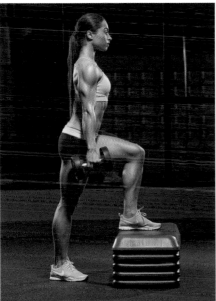

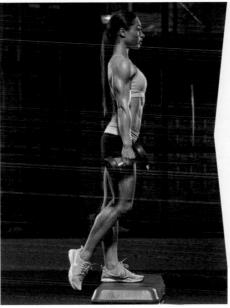

BENCH STEP-UP

• Grasp a dumbbell in each hand and stand behind the center of a weight bench or step.

• Hold your arms straight down at your sides with your palms facing inward; keep your shoulders relaxed, back, and down.

• Place your left foot firmly on top of the bench or step so that your left knee is bent and aligned directly over your ankle.

• Slightly bend your right knee and push off the floor to lift yourself upward.

• Pause briefly at the top and then step your right leg back down to the start.

• Complete reps with the left leg and then switch legs and repeat.

SATURDAY
Breakfast
3 egg whites, scrambled or boiled
1 tbsp flaxseeds
½ cup oat bran
Late-morning Snack
3 oz chicken breast, white meat
¾ oz English walnuts, halves

Lunch
½ cup zucchini
4 oz chicken breast, white meat
2 soft corn tortillas, 7-inch diameter
Midday Snack
½ medium banana
1 tbsp flaxseeds
3 egg whites, scrambled or boiled

Dinner
1 oz avocado
1½ cups baby spinach
4 oz turkey breast, white meat
Nighttime Snack
1 tbsp almond butter, natural
1½ scoops whey protein
TOTALS: 1,483 Calories, 179g Protein, 91g Carbs, 51g Fat

SUNDAY
Breakfast
3 egg whites, scrambled or boiled
1 tbsp flaxseeds
⅓ cup oatmeal, quick, measured uncooked
Late-morning Snack
3 oz chicken breast, white meat
¾ oz English walnuts, halves

Lunch
4 oz green beans
4 oz tilapia
½ cup brown rice
Midday Snack
½ medium apple
1 tbsp flaxseeds
1½ scoops whey protein
Dinner
1 oz avocado
4 oz asparagus
3 egg whites, scrambled

or boiled
Nighttime Snack
1 tbsp peanut butter, natural
1½ scoops whey protein
TOTALS: 1,410 Calories, 164g Protein, 88g Carbs, 42g Fat

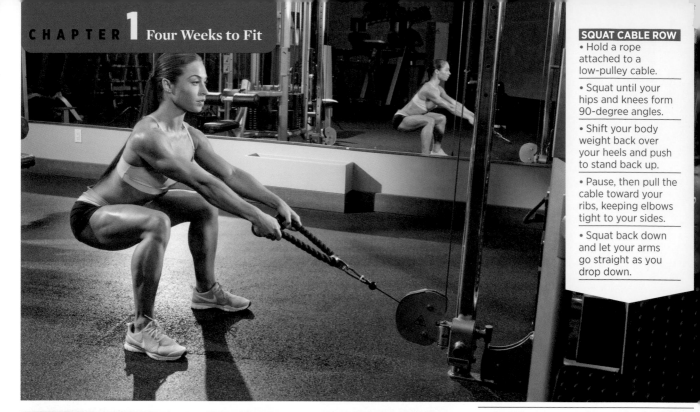

SQUAT CABLE ROW
- Hold a rope attached to a low-pulley cable.
- Squat until your hips and knees form 90-degree angles.
- Shift your body weight back over your heels and push to stand back up.
- Pause, then pull the cable toward your ribs, keeping elbows tight to your sides.
- Squat back down and let your arms go straight as you drop down.

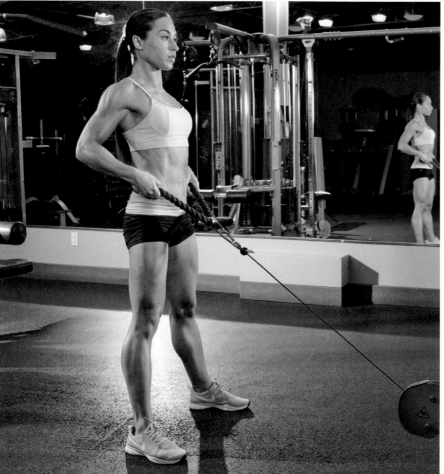

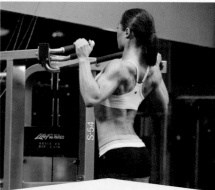

MACHINE-ASSISTED PULLUP
- Take an overhand grip on the bar of a pullup machine.
- Fully extend your arms and relax your shoulders to stretch your lats.
- Squeeze your shoulder blades together, arch your back, focus on your lats, and pull your body up, aiming your chest toward the bar.
- Pull yourself up until your chin is level with or slightly above the bar.
- Hold the top position momentarily, then lower your body under control back to the starting position.
- Repeat for reps.

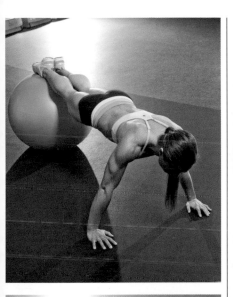

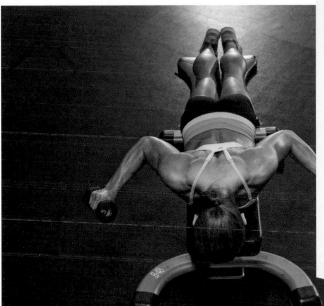

SHOULDER YTWL CIRCUIT

• Lie facedown on a flat bench, arms extended forward in a Y position, palms facing the floor.

• Lower arms into a T position, then bend at the elbows and draw upper arms down 45 degrees to the torso, forming a W.

• Keeping your upper arms at your sides and palms facing the floor, lower forearms to form an L (not shown), then push arms back to start position and repeat.

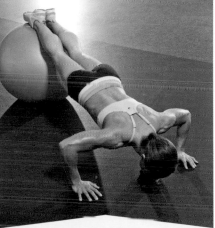

EXERCISE BALL PUSHUP

• Lying facedown on an exercise ball, place your hands on the floor in front of you.

• Walk your hands forward, rolling the ball underneath you until you're balanced with the ball under your shins and ankles.

• Keep your legs together, arms extended with fingertips facing forward and your hands slightly wider than your shoulders.

• Contract your abs, drawing your tailbone down so your body forms a straight line from head to heels in plank position.

• Maintain plank and bend your elbows, lowering your chest toward the floor until elbows are in line with shoulders; keep your wrists aligned under your elbows with forearms parallel to each other.

• Press back up to the starting position and repeat.

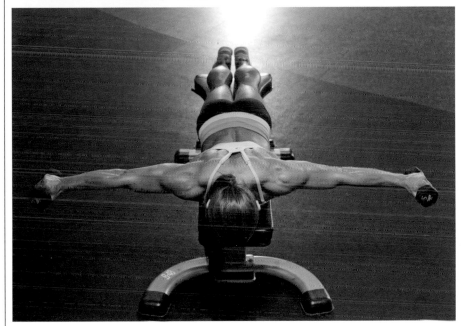

Upper-Body Plyometrics Workout (Day 4)

EXERCISE	Circuit 1* REPS	Circuit 2* REPS	Circuit 3* REPS	Circuit 4* REPS
Exercise Ball Pushup	15	12	10	8
Overhead Medicine Ball Throw	15	12	10	8
Machine Assisted Pullup	12	10	8	8
Squat Cable Row	15	10	8	8
Shoulder YTWL Circuit	20	15	12	10

*Between each circuit, complete five minutes on treadmill, StepMill, or elliptical at 70–75% MHR.

Lift
LIKE A
Girl

Build the body you've always wanted with these five no-nonsense moves

Many women are terrified of putting on muscle. But as anyone who has been in the gym longer than three months knows, it just isn't that easy. It's safe to say, however, that the majority of *Hers* readers want to do exactly that—add shape in all the right places. After all, strategically placed muscle will only enhance your appearance, giving you curves right where you've always wanted them. Plus, you'll have that highly sought-after tight and toned look.

With that in mind, we've broken down five basic, hardcore exercises we guarantee you won't see at your neighborhood Curves. Since these free-weight, compound moves are designed to help you add the muscle you want, you'll use slightly lower rep ranges—as low as six and as high as 10—for each. To make sure you get it right, we enlisted the help of *Hers* senior science editor, Jim Stoppani, Ph.D., to break down all the do's, don'ts, and insider tips you'll need to make the fab five work for you. They could be the difference between wanting the body of your dreams and having it.

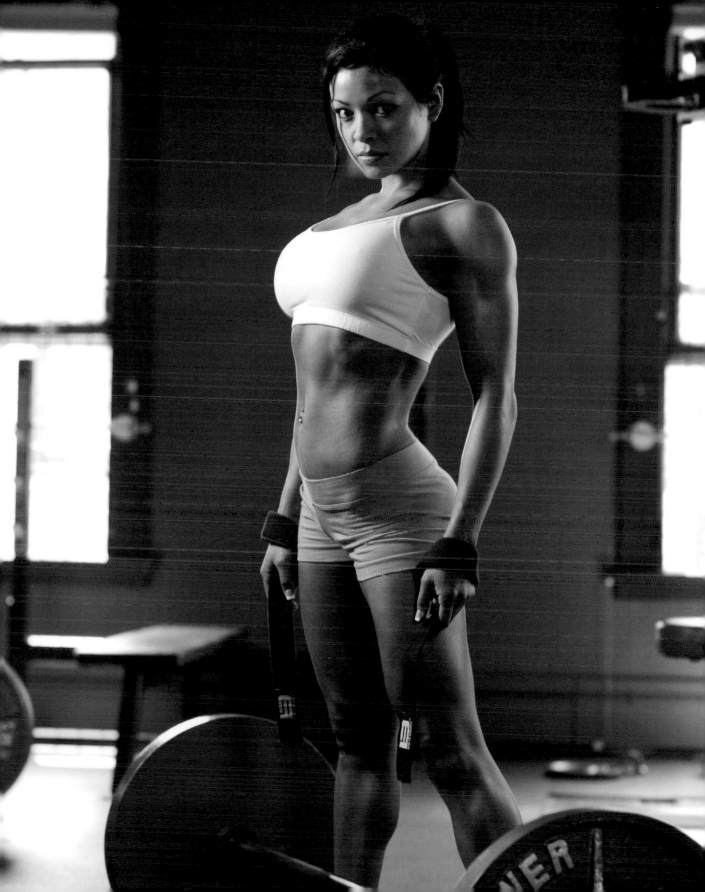

Split Like a Girl

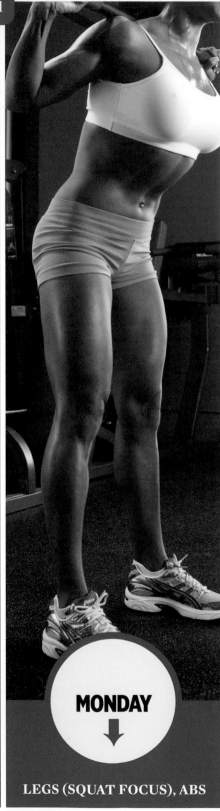

MONDAY
⬇

LEGS (SQUAT FOCUS), ABS

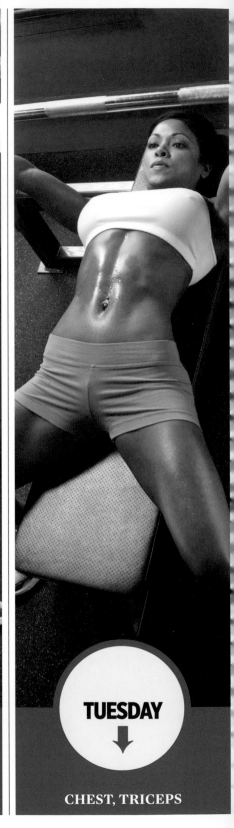

TUESDAY
⬇

CHEST, TRICEPS

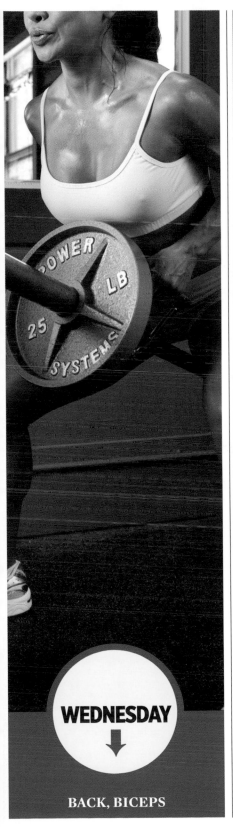

WEDNESDAY
↓

BACK, BICEPS

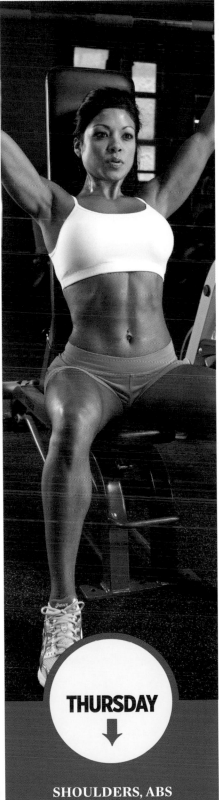

THURSDAY
↓

SHOULDERS, ABS

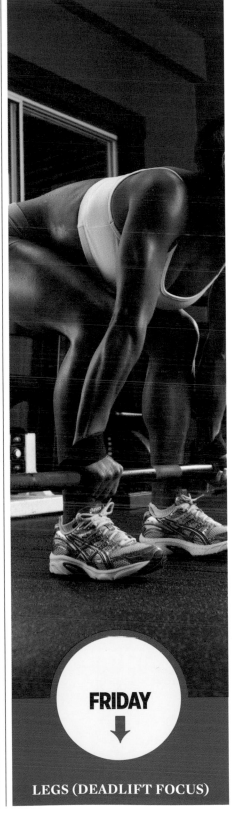

FRIDAY
↓

LEGS (DEADLIFT FOCUS)

Seated Overhead Press

MAJOR MUSCLES WORKED
• Front deltoids, middle deltoids
SECONDARY MUSCLES
• Trapezius, triceps

The most basic and effective exercise for building impressive shoulders, this move should be the anchor of your deltoid routine. Strong, shapely shoulders are the cornerstones of an eye-pleasing physique and are sure to make your waistline appear smaller for a more pronounced hourglass figure.

FORM & FUNCTION
The shoulder, or deltoid, is made up of three heads—anterior, middle, and posterior. The anterior (front) head moves the arm forward and across the body at the shoulder joint. The middle head moves the arm outward and upward. The posterior (rear) head extends the arm backward at the shoulder joint.

WHEN TO PRESS
Because the seated overhead press works the entire shoulder area, do it first in your workout when your strength levels are highest. Follow with another multijoint, free-weight movement like upright rows, then isolation moves like cable lateral raises for the middle deltoids and dumbbell bentover lateral raises for the rear delts.

Sample Shoulder Routine

EXERCISE	SETS	REPS
Seated Overhead Press	3	6–10
Dumbbell Upright Row	3	8–12
Cable Lateral Raise	3	10–12
Dumbbell Bentover Lateral Raise	3	12–15

• Hold the bar in line with your clavicles, with your elbows close to your sides. Keep your lower back tight, upper back arched, chest out, and head tilted back slightly with your chin up.

• Grasp the bar with your thumbs wrapped around it, hands slightly wider than shoulder width. An excessively wide grip will overly stress your elbows and wrists; an excessively narrow grip will shift the emphasis from your delts to your triceps.

• Keep your lower back flat against the bench and as erect as possible. If your glutes scoot forward, you'll stress more of the upper chest and less of the deltoids.

• Inhale and hold your breath. Keeping your upper body stable, push the bar straight overhead.

• Keep your feet anchored flat on the floor, shoulder-width apart or slightly wider, to provide a solid base of power.

• As the bar ascends, move your elbows out to your sides to put more stress on the middle deltoids.

• Stop just short of full-arm extension to keep the stress on your delts.

• Exhale and slowly lower the bar to the start position, focusing on your shoulders.

• Most gyms are equipped with an overhead-press bench with a rack, but if yours isn't, select a bench with a back support and place it in front of a power rack or squat rack. Be sure the bench is far enough away that you don't hit the uprights as you press the bar but close enough that you can get the bar out of the rack comfortably.

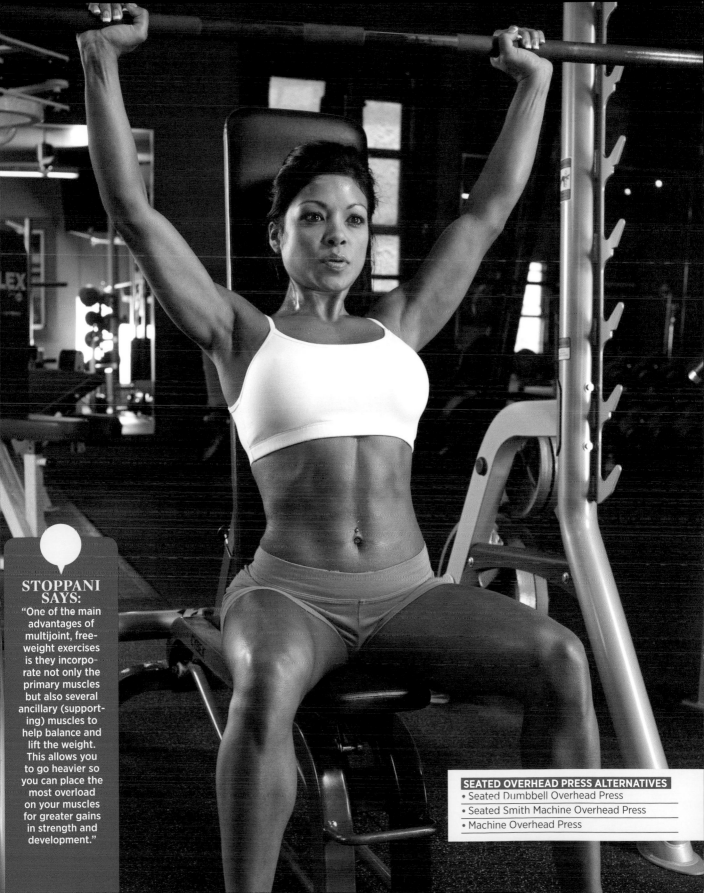

SEATED OVERHEAD PRESS ALTERNATIVES
• Seated Dumbbell Overhead Press
• Seated Smith Machine Overhead Press
• Machine Overhead Press

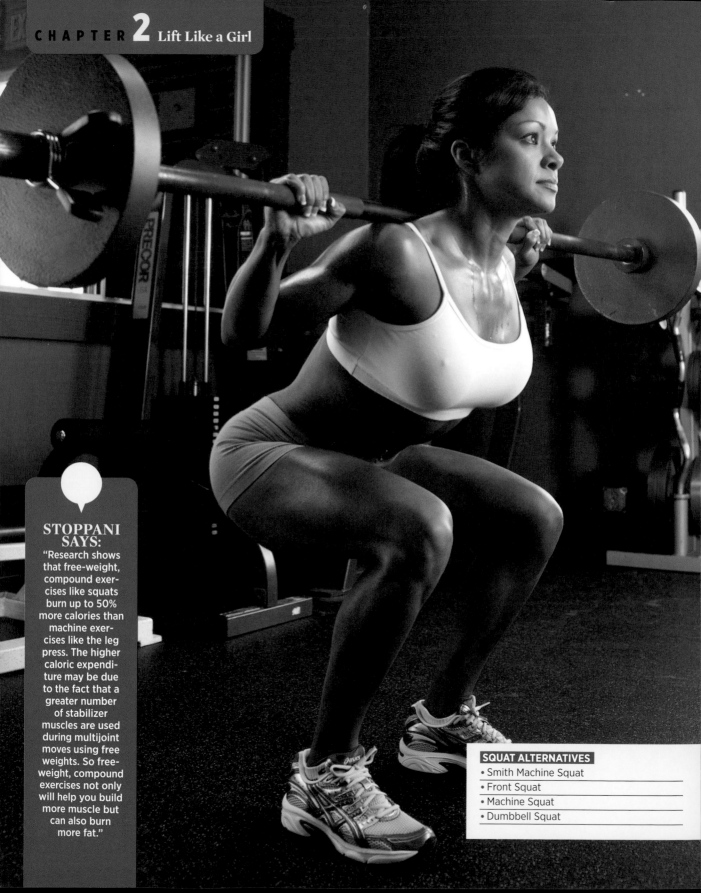

STOPPANI SAYS:

"Research shows that free-weight, compound exercises like squats burn up to 50% more calories than machine exercises like the leg press. The higher caloric expenditure may be due to the fact that a greater number of stabilizer muscles are used during multijoint moves using free weights. So free-weight, compound exercises not only will help you build more muscle but can also burn more fat."

SQUAT ALTERNATIVES
- Smith Machine Squat
- Front Squat
- Machine Squat
- Dumbbell Squat

Squat

MAJOR MUSCLES WORKED
• Quadriceps, hamstrings, glutes
SECONDARY MUSCLES
• Calves, erector spinae, abs

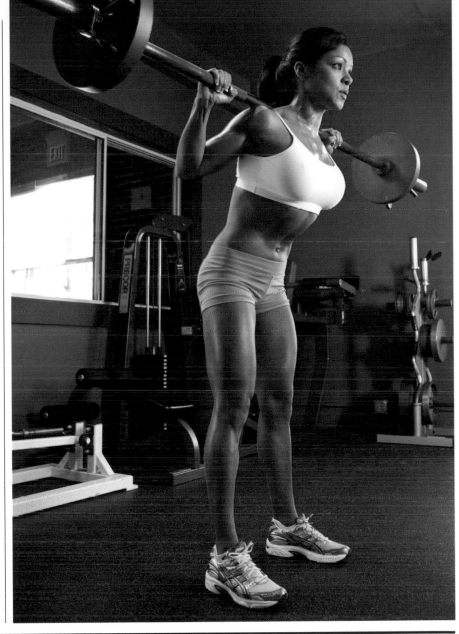

The squat is the queen of lower-body exercises, and nothing else will do more to get your lower half in tip-top shape. Since it hits every major muscle group in the lower body, squatting will ensure your legs look great from every angle. Strong legs are also critical for most sports and athletic activities.

FORM & FUNCTION
The quadriceps is composed of the vastus lateralis (outside), vastus medialis (inside), rectus femoris (middle upper), and vastus intermedius (under the rectus femoris). The hamstring on the back of the thigh is composed of the biceps femoris (outside), semitendinosus (inside), and semimembranosus (under the semitendinosus). The gluteus maximus extends the hip and helps turn the thigh outward.

WHEN TO SQUAT
Since the squat requires a great deal of strength and energy to perform correctly, tackle it first in your workout. Follow with another multijoint exercise like the leg press before doing isolation movements, for optimal leg development.

Sample Leg Routine (SQUAT FOCUS)

EXERCISE	SETS	REPS
Squat	3	6–10
Leg Press	3	8 12
Leg Extension	3	12–15
Romanian Deadlift	3	8–12
Lying Leg Curl	3	12–15

• Grasping the bar with your thumbs wrapped around it, bring your hands as close to your shoulders as possible and press the bar against your back. Squeezing your shoulder blades together and pulling your elbows forward will help you support the bar.

• Keep your head aligned with your spine by fixing your gaze on an object at eye level.

• Maintain the arch in your lower back, and push your chest up and out. Contract your spinal erector muscles and abs to keep your core tight.

• The bar should rest near your mid-traps and rear delts (rather than your upper traps). This will make it easier to balance the weight throughout the exercise.

• Keep a slight bend in your knees, and contract your quads, hamstrings, and glutes. Take a deep breath and hold it as you begin your descent.

• Place your feet just wider than shoulder width, though this will vary slightly depending on flexibility and comfort.

• Without lifting your chin, push your head back to help contract your traps for greater stability.

• Concentrate on moving your hips before bending your knees. Keep your hips under the bar as much as possible to avoid leaning forward. This will relieve stress on your lower back.

• Your knees should never pass your toes, to avoid placing a dangerous amount of stress on your knee joints.

• Push your glutes out as if sitting in a chair. Descend until your thighs are slightly below parallel to the floor.

• As you ascend, force your knees out hard and push out on the sides of your shoes. This will help keep tension in your hips for greater strength.

• Keep your heels on the floor to avoid leaning forward.

Bench Press

MAJOR MUSCLES WORKED
• Pectoralis major
SECONDARY MUSCLES
• Deltoids, triceps, latissimus dorsi

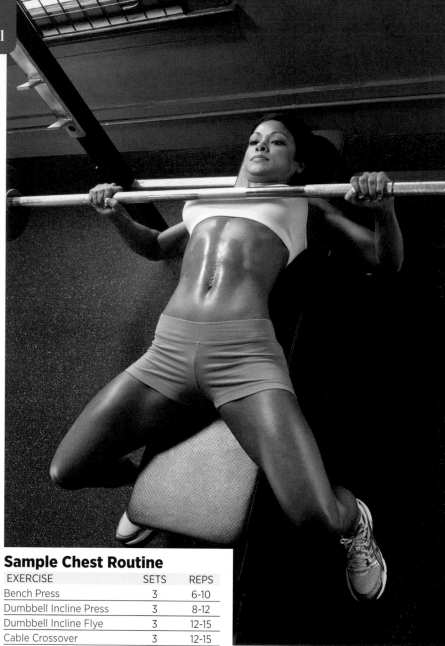

Want to look great from the front? A shapely chest is the centerpiece, and this do-it-all upper-body exercise that also targets your shoulders and triceps will sculpt muscle like no other. This enhances your athletic appearance and functional upper-body strength.

FORM & FUNCTION

The pectoralis major (pecs) makes up the chest and is composed of two distinct heads that start at different areas of the torso but converge onto the same tendon. The clavicular head (upper pecs) starts on the clavicle or collarbone; the sternocostal head (middle and lower pecs) starts on the sternum and ribs. Both heads meet via a tendon that attaches to the humerus (upper arm bone), and work to adduct and flex the arm at the shoulder, as in the bench press.

WHEN TO BENCH

Do it first in your chest workout to target the entire pectoral area. Since the upper chest shows most on women, progress to two exercises that hit this area—incline presses and an isolation exercise like incline flyes. Finish with cable crossovers, another isolation exercise, to enhance shape.

Sample Chest Routine

EXERCISE	SETS	REPS
Bench Press	3	6-10
Dumbbell Incline Press	3	8-12
Dumbbell Incline Flye	3	12-15
Cable Crossover	3	12-15

• Take a slightly wider than shoulder-width grip on the bar. Wrap your thumbs around it to prevent flexing your wrists back too much, which could decrease force production traveling through the forearm and overall strength.

• Hold the bar over your upper chest. Inhale deeply and hold it as you descend. This increases pressure in your chest and abdominal cavity for added support and force production.

• Maintain a slight arch in your lower back throughout the exercise, and keep your shoulders and glutes pressed into the bench for stability.

• Lie faceup on the bench with your feet flat on the floor and wider than shoulder-width apart, toes pointed out. Your knees should be bent at about 90-degree angles.

• Press the bar straight up, trying to move it as quickly as possible. Although it'll move slowly, the resulting neural drive will recruit more fast-twitch muscle fibers, the ones most responsible for muscle size and strength.

• Squeeze the bar as hard as you can to transmit force from your chest, shoulders, and triceps to the bar. Try to rip the bar apart by pulling your arms out without changing your grip.

• Exhale as you pass the most difficult part of the lift.

• Contract your chest muscles, stopping just short of full-arm extension to keep tension on the pecs.

• Imagining the bar is empty, explode the weight off your chest by driving your heels into the floor to transfer force to your upper body. Keep your glutes on the bench.

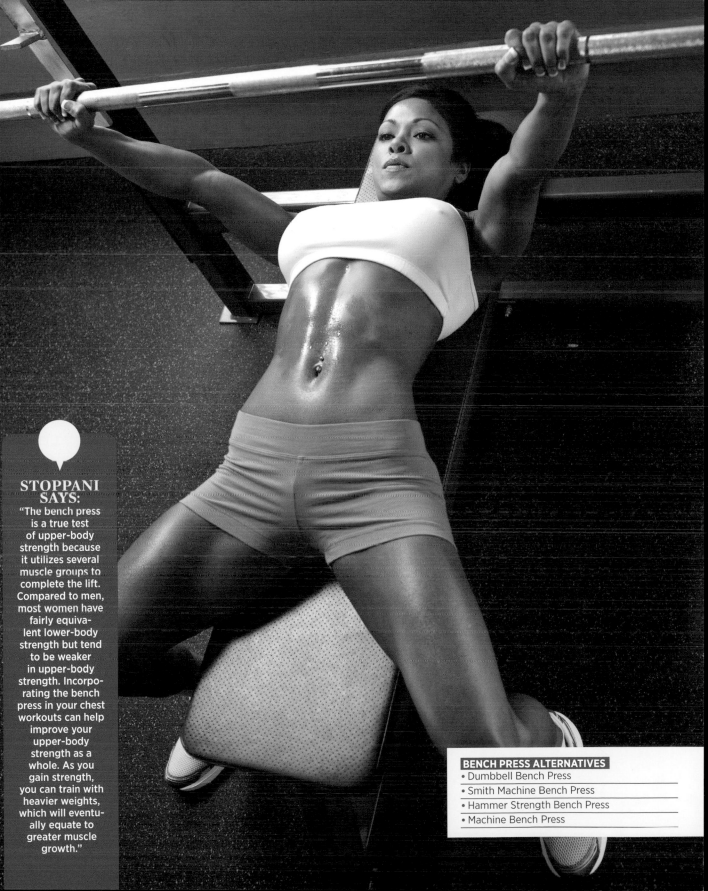

STOPPANI SAYS:

"The bench press is a true test of upper-body strength because it utilizes several muscle groups to complete the lift. Compared to men, most women have fairly equivalent lower-body strength but tend to be weaker in upper-body strength. Incorporating the bench press in your chest workouts can help improve your upper-body strength as a whole. As you gain strength, you can train with heavier weights, which will eventually equate to greater muscle growth."

BENCH PRESS ALTERNATIVES
• Dumbbell Bench Press
• Smith Machine Bench Press
• Hammer Strength Bench Press
• Machine Bench Press

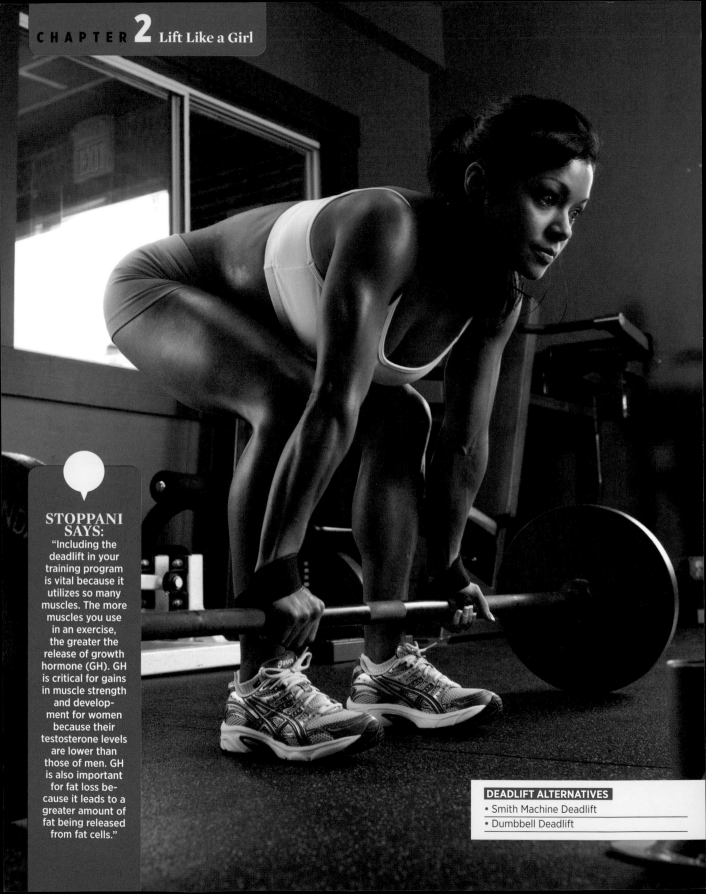

STOPPANI SAYS:
"Including the deadlift in your training program is vital because it utilizes so many muscles. The more muscles you use in an exercise, the greater the release of growth hormone (GH). GH is critical for gains in muscle strength and development for women because their testosterone levels are lower than those of men. GH is also important for fat loss because it leads to a greater amount of fat being released from fat cells."

DEADLIFT ALTERNATIVES
- Smith Machine Deadlift
- Dumbbell Deadlift

Deadlift

MAJOR MUSCLES WORKED
• Quadriceps, hamstrings, erector spinae, gluteus maximus

SECONDARY MUSCLES
• Latissimus dorsi, rhomboids, teres major, trapezius, forearms, abs

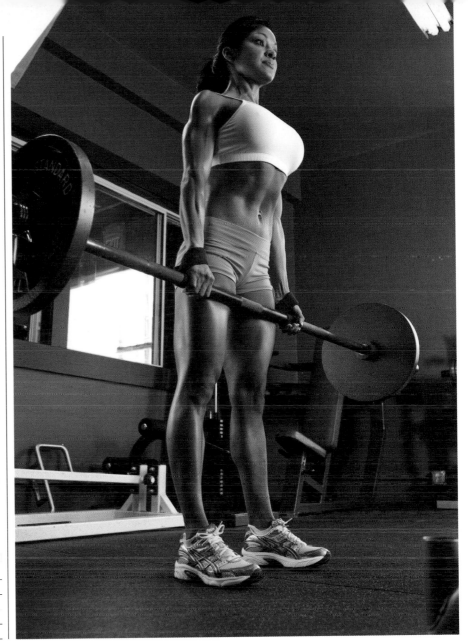

There's a reason why the deadlift is considered a superior exercise: This total-body blast works almost every muscle in the body from head to toe. It's tough and can take a lot out of you, but master this exercise and you can have the legs, glutes, back and everything else you've always wanted.

FORM & FUNCTION
The deadlift mimics the squat in several ways, but because you hold the bar in front of your body, the hamstrings, glutes, and erector spinae play a more critical role than the quads. The erector spinae is a group of muscles that run along the spine and extend it.

WHEN TO DEADLIFT
While the deadlift involves the lower back and other back muscles to some degree, it primarily targets the hams, glutes, and quads. Therefore, it's best to include deadlifts on leg day. One of the best methods is to train legs twice a week. In one leg workout do deadlifts as your first exercise, and in the second do squats as your first move. This way you'll get the benefits of two of the very best lower-body exercises ever.

Sample Leg Routine
(DEADLIFT FOCUS)

EXERCISE	SETS	REPS
Deadlift	4	6 10
Front Squat	3	8–12
Leg Extension	3	12–15
Romanian Deadlift	3	8–12
Seated Leg Curl	3	12–15

• To keep your head in a straight line with your back, focus on a point on the floor 5–6 feet in front of you.

• Contract your lower-back muscles to maintain the natural arch in your spine. Keep your shoulder blades pulled together tightly throughout the exercise.

• Keep your abs pulled in tightly throughout the lift.

• Bend your knees so your thighs are slightly above parallel to the floor and lean forward at the hips so your torso is at about a 45-degree angle to the floor. Most of your weight should be distributed over your heels to maximize the contribution of the hamstrings and glutes.

• Your arms should hang straight down just outside your thighs. The bar should touch your shins.

• Use an alternate grip—one underhand grip and one overhand grip—for maximal strength and minimal bar slippage.

• Your feet should be about shoulder-width apart or closer, toes pointed straight ahead or slightly outward (25 degrees, at most).

• Exhale as you reach the top position. Descend slowly, "tapping" the weights to the floor.

• Your hips and shoulders should rise together for maximal power output. Don't lead with your glutes, which could place a great deal of stress on your lower back.

• Fully extend your knees, hips, and back, keeping the front of your shoulders behind the front of your hips.

• As you begin the ascent, exert a small amount of upward force on the bar before pulling it up. Drive down with your heels and imagine that you're pushing the floor away.

• Keep the bar as close to your shins and legs as possible to avoid leaning forward, which would diminish power and could result in serious injury to your lower back.

T-Bar Row

MAJOR MUSCLES WORKED
- Latissimus dorsi, teres major

SECONDARY MUSCLES
- Rear deltoids, rhomboids, trapezius

Forget those nice, comfy machines; we're going old-school here. Sure, it's a little more work, but there's a reason this standby has been around for so long: It delivers results. A well-developed back will create the illusion of a smaller waist to accentuate the shape of your body and improve your posture.

FORM & FUNCTION

The latissimus dorsi (lats) starts on the seventh thoracic vertebra and goes all the way down to the sacrum and rear portion of the hipbone. The upper-lat fibers cover the thoracic spine down to about the bottom of the lumbar spine, while the lower-lat fibers cover the sacrum and hipbone. Both sections converge onto the same tendon that attaches to the humerus and help pull the arm toward the ribs via extension and adduction.

WHEN TO T-BAR ROW

Do it at the start of your workout when your back muscles are strongest. This will allow you to use heavier weight and place more overload on your lats. Follow T-bar rows with pulldowns as well as other rowing exercises. Finish your workout with an isolation movement.

Sample Back Routine

EXERCISE	SETS	REPS
T-bar Row	3	6–10
Wide-grip Lat Pulldown	3	8–12
Seated Cable Row	3	8–12
Straight-arm Pulldown	3	12–15

- Place one end of an empty bar in a corner with a 45-pound weight plate on top to keep it from moving. This will act as the pivot point. Slide weight plates onto the opposite end but don't use anything heavier than 25-pounders. Larger plates will impede the range of motion.

- Secure a V-bar handle under the weighted end of the bar, as close to the collar as possible. If necessary, use straps to assist your grip so your biceps and forearms don't give out before your back is fully fatigued.

- Place your feet flat on the floor, shoulder-width apart. Bend your knees to about 45-degree angles.

- Moving only your arms, concentrate on pulling with your lats as you drive your elbows back. Keep your elbows in tight to your sides to fully engage your lats and other back muscles.

- Keep your back arched as you reach the top position. Squeeze your lats tightly.

- Pull the handle toward your abs to work your entire back.

- Lean forward at the hips so your torso is between parallel and less than a 45-degree angle to the floor.

- Keep your head in line with your back by focusing on a spot on the floor slightly in front of you. Pull your shoulders back, and arch your lower back.

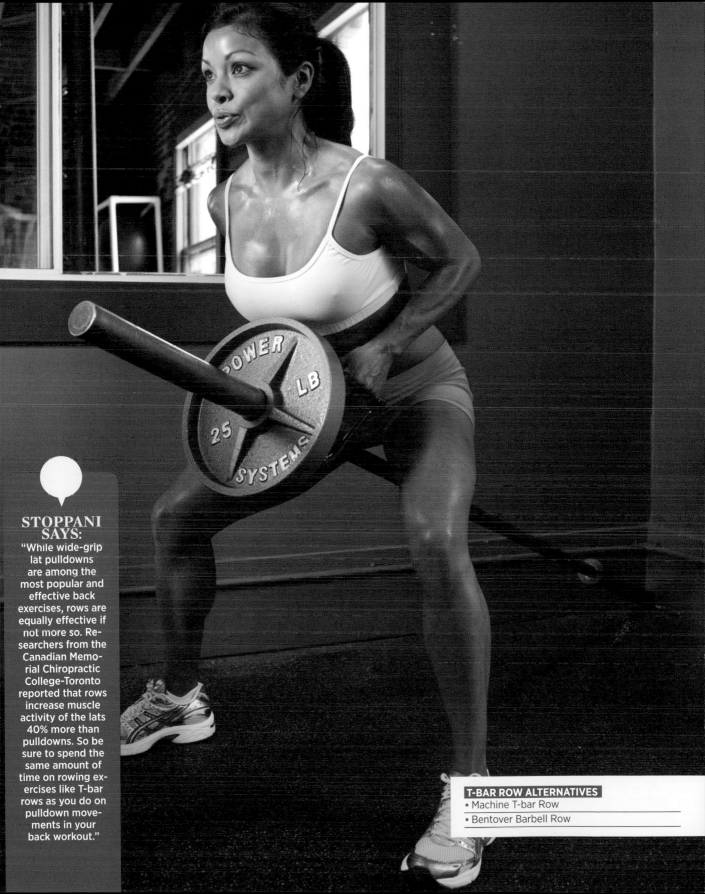

STOPPANI SAYS:

"While wide-grlp lat pulldowns are among the most popular and effective back exercises, rows are equally effective if not more so. Researchers from the Canadian Memorial Chiropractic College-Toronto reported that rows increase muscle activity of the lats 40% more than pulldowns. So be sure to spend the same amount of time on rowing exercises like T-bar rows as you do on pulldown movements in your back workout."

T-BAR ROW ALTERNATIVES
• Machine T-bar Row
• Bentover Barbell Row

CHAPTER 3

RESULTS, Period

Adopt a specific plan—like periodization training—for your regimen to promote long-term results and avoid plateaus

It's about time we stepped in and intervened, because far too many people have become far too predictable in their training habits. Walk into any standard gym or health club in the country and we can almost guarantee that the majority of people working out there — from newbies to hardcore fitness junkies — will be training in the exact manner six months down the road. Same exercises. Same rep ranges. Same volume. Same weights. And, unfortunately, same results.

Want to start getting better results? Then it's time to devise a plan. It's time for a big, scientific-sounding word with a bunch of syllables that, in practice, is far less intimidating than it looks on paper. It's time for periodization, people.

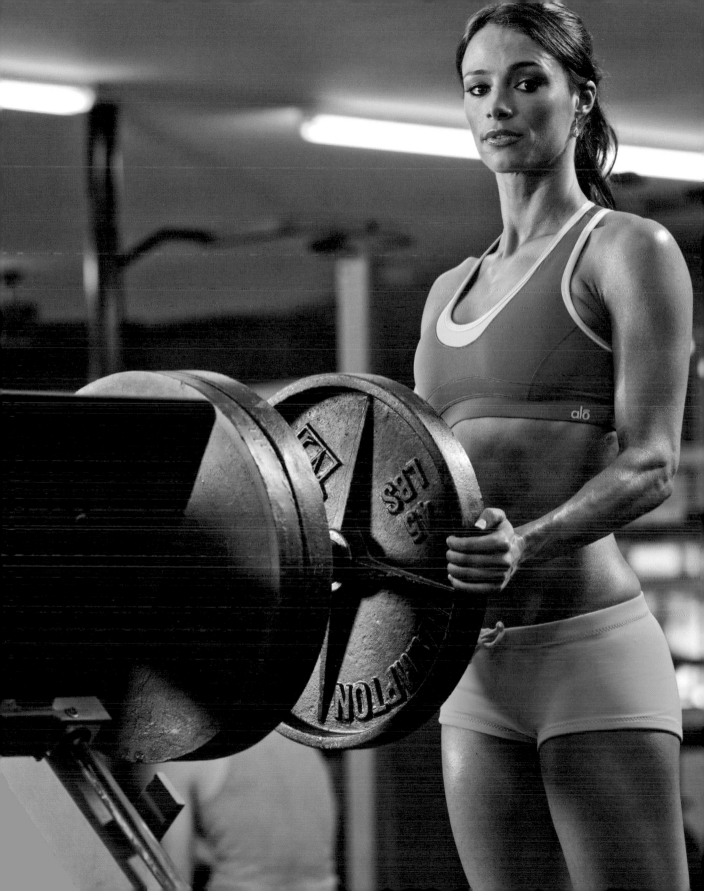

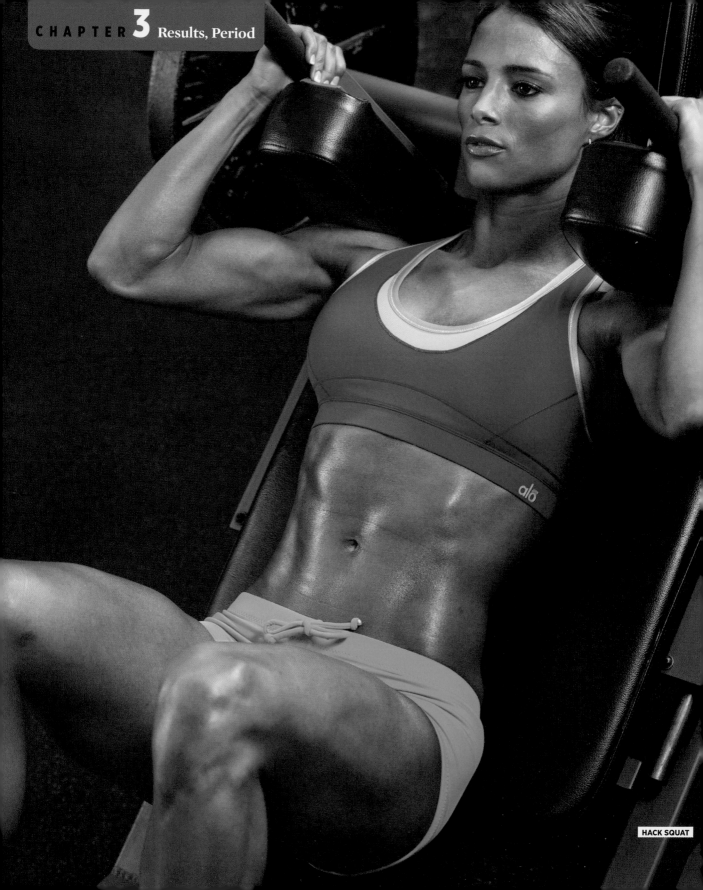

HACK SQUAT

Periodization Primer

"Periodization" refers to the manipulation of training variables—weight used, reps completed, exercises selected, rest periods between sets—over a period of days, months, or years. The original concept was developed in the former Eastern Bloc countries in the late 1950s to enhance athletes' performance in the gym and on playing fields. Periodization typically revolves around an athlete's competitive calendar, allowing him or her to "peak" for competition—whether that competition is a triathlon, an important swim meet, or even a figure contest.

The basis behind periodization is a concept called the general adaptation syndrome, which involves three stages that an athlete goes through when exposed to a new type of training:

1) As a new stress is placed on the body—let's use heavy training in the three- to five-rep range as an example—the muscle first goes through an alarm reaction and the individual actually gets weaker. But not for long.

2) Soon enough, with successive workouts, the body begins to adapt. In this adaptation stage, the body typically compensates by increasing muscle strength to better deal with the new stress. This is a good thing, of course, but if the body is continually exposed to the training style for too long, it can enter a stage of exhaustion where strength levels not only plateau but actually decrease.

3) The trick is to expose the body to a particular style of training just long enough for it to adapt and get stronger, but not so long that it becomes counterproductive and leads to decreased performance or, worse, injury. In a perfect world, just as the body is about to stop showing improvement, you'd introduce yet another new training style and the cycle of adaptation would repeat itself.

Admittedly, this is a very simplistic take on periodization, and the "perfect world" scenario is way easier said than done, but you get the idea.

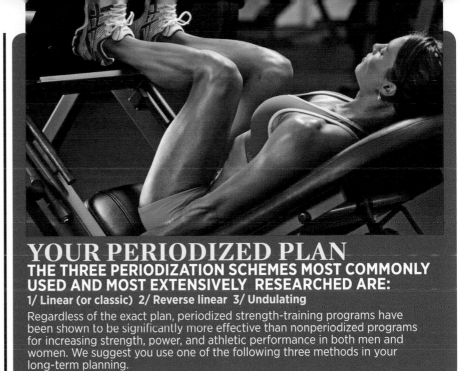

YOUR PERIODIZED PLAN
THE THREE PERIODIZATION SCHEMES MOST COMMONLY USED AND MOST EXTENSIVELY RESEARCHED ARE:
1/ Linear (or classic) 2/ Reverse linear 3/ Undulating

Regardless of the exact plan, periodized strength-training programs have been shown to be significantly more effective than nonperiodized programs for increasing strength, power, and athletic performance in both men and women. We suggest you use one of the following three methods in your long-term planning.

LINEAR PERIODIZATION

This is the scheme that more or less started the whole periodization revolution. In its simplest form, a linear periodized program progresses from light weight done for high reps (about 12–15, but sometimes 20 or more reps) to heavy weight done for low reps (anywhere from 1 to 5 reps per set).

The original linear plan included six different phases, where rep ranges descended in the following fashion: 1) general preparedness phase (around 15 reps per set); 2) hypertrophy (8–12); 3) strength (3–6); 4) power (2–3); 5) peaking (1–3, with fewer total sets); and, finally, 6) active rest, where practically no strength-training was done at all.

But if you're not a world-class athlete preparing for competition, the original approach is probably not a good fit for you. That's not to say that you can't glean valuable points from it to accelerate your gains in the gym. The best way to use the linear periodization model is to break it down into four phases:

Week 1:
Light weight for 12–15 reps per set

Week 2:
Weights increase and reps drop down to 9–11

Week 3:
Weight increases again to bring reps down to 6–8

Week 4:
Weight increases yet again with reps dropping to just 3–5 per set

At right is one example of this form of linear periodized training. Give it a try to achieve a stronger, tighter, more athletic pair of legs.

4-WEEK LINEAR PERIODIZATION FOR LEGS

EXERCISE	SETS/REPS	REST
WEEK 1		
Hack Squat	4/12–15	1 min.
Dumbbell Lunge	3/12–15	1 min.
Leg Press	3/12–15	1 min.
Leg Extension	3/12–15	1 min.
Leg Curl	3/12–15	1 min.
WEEK 2		
Hack Squat	4/9–11	90–120 sec.
Dumbbell Lunge	3/9–11	90–120 sec.
Leg Press	3/9–11	90–120 sec.
Leg Extension	3/9–11	90–120 sec.
Leg Curl	3/9–11	90–120 sec.

EXERCISE	SETS/REPS	REST
WEEK 3		
Hack Squat	4/6–8	2–3 min.
Dumbbell Lunge	3/6–8	2–3 min.
Leg Press	3/6–8	2–3 min.
Leg Extension	3/6–8	2–3 min.
Leg Curl	3/6–8	2–3 min.
WEEK 4		
Hack Squat	4/3–5	3 min.
Dumbbell Lunge	3/3–5	3 min.
Leg Press	3/3–5	3 min.
Leg Extension	3/3–5	3 min.
Leg Curl	3/3–5	3 min.

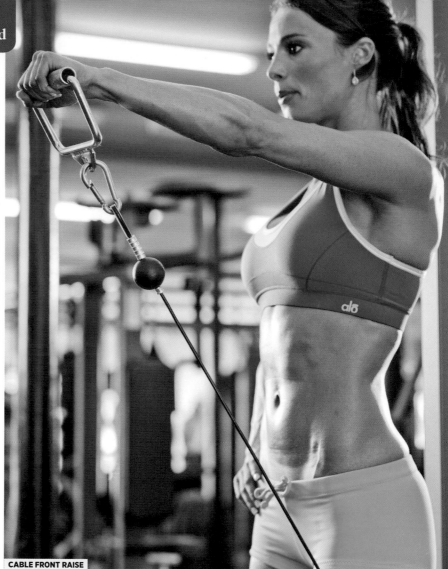

CABLE FRONT RAISE

REVERSE LINEAR PERIODIZATION

Reverse linear periodization basically takes the linear (classic) periodization scheme and runs it backward. While the goal of the classic periodization model is typically to maximize an athlete's strength and power, the goal of the reverse linear model is to maximize muscle hypertrophy or endurance strength—depending on the rep range that the program concludes with (10–15 reps for hypertrophy or 20–30+ reps for endurance strength). Research supports the concept that the reverse linear periodization scheme is more effective for increasing endurance strength than the linear model.

An example of a four-week reverse linear periodization program would look like this:

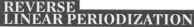

Week 1:
Heavy weights, low reps (3–5 per set)
Week 2:
Weight decreases slightly, 6–8 reps per set
Week 3:
Weight decreases again, reps raised to 9–11
Week 4:
Weight decreases again, reps increased to 12–15 per set

At right is a sample program for shoulders. The objective is hypertrophy, evidenced by the fact that in the final week the rep counts are 12–15. Use this plan for the next month if your goal is to add muscle to your delts for a more shapely, appealing upper body.

4-WEEK REVERSE LINEAR PERIODIZATION FOR SHOULDERS

EXERCISE	SETS/REPS	REST
WEEK 1		
Dumbbell Shoulder Press	3/3–5	3 min.
Smith Machine Upright Row	3/3–5	3 min.
Dumbbell Lateral Raise	3/3–5	3 min.
Cable Front Raise	2/3–5	3 min.
Reverse Machine Flye	2/3–5	3 min.
WEEK 2		
Dumbbell Shoulder Press	3/6–8	2–3 min.
Smith Machine Upright Row	3/6–8	2–3 min.
Dumbbell Lateral Raise	3/6–8	2–3 min.
Cable Front Raise	2/6–8	2–3 min.
Reverse Machine Flye	2/6–8	2–3 min.

EXERCISE	SETS/REPS	REST
WEEK 3		
Dumbbell Shoulder Press	3/9–11	90–120 sec.
Smith Machine Upright Rows	3/9–11	90–120 sec.
Dumbbell Lateral Raise	3/9–11	90–120 sec.
Cable Front Raise	2/9–11	90–120 sec.
Reverse Machine Flye	2/9–11	90–120 sec.
WEEK 4		
Dumbbell Shoulder Press	3/12–15	1 min.
Smith Machine Upright Row	3/12–15	1 min.
Dumbbell Lateral Raise	3/12–15	1 min.
Cable Front Raise	2/12–15	1 min.
Reverse Machine Flye	2/12–15	1 min.

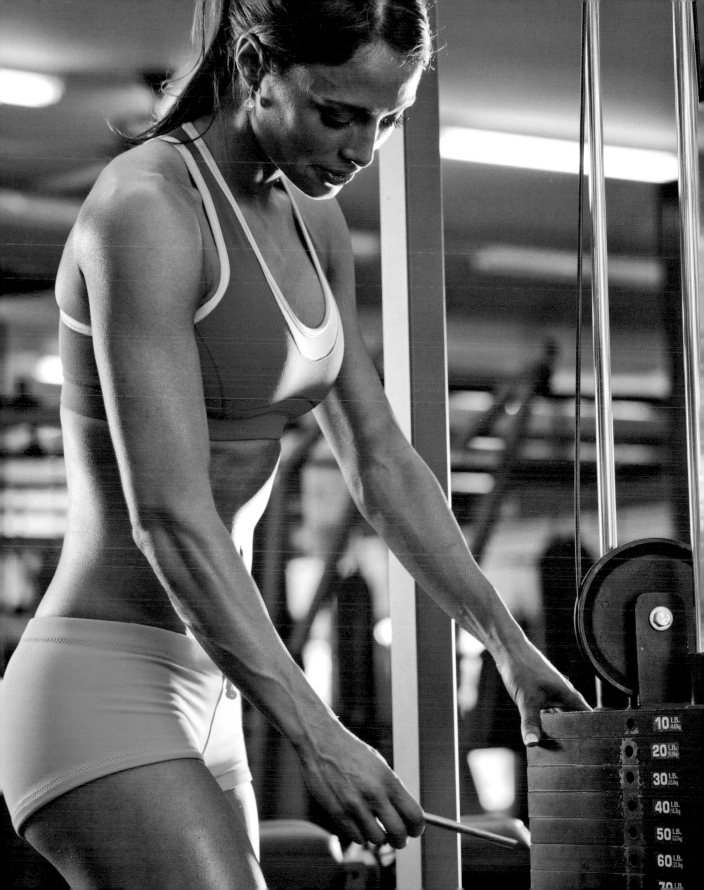

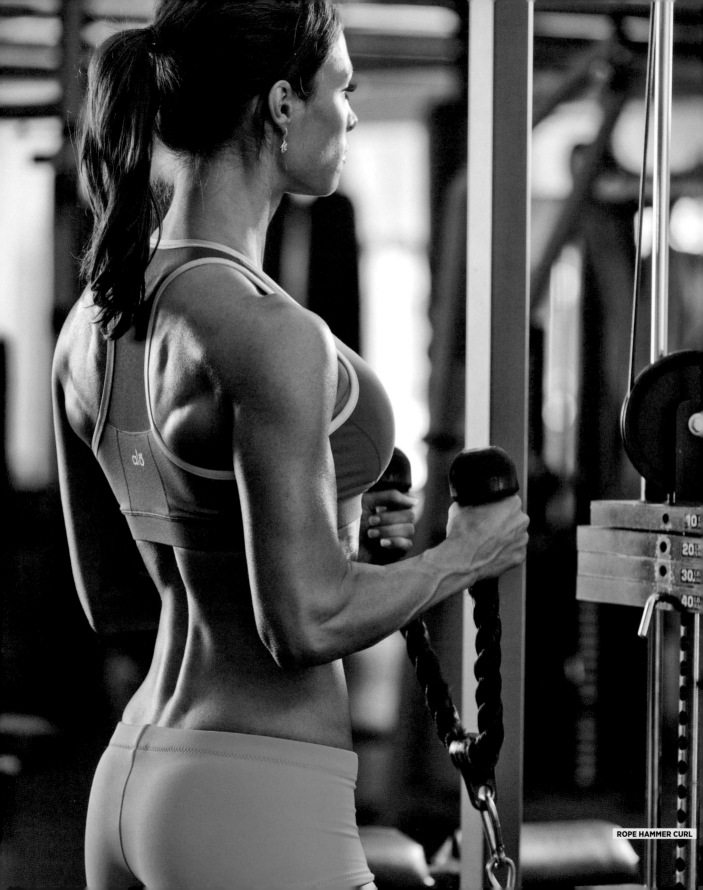

ROPE HAMMER CURL

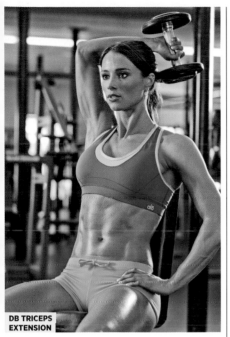

DB TRICEPS EXTENSION

UNDULATING PERIODIZATION

Undulating periodization is just a fancy way of saying "muscle confusion." While linear and reverse linear protocols gradually increase or decrease the weight, undulating calls for the weight and rep ranges to jump all over the place, with different weights and rep ranges virtually every workout.

Some days you go heavy with low reps, other days you go light with high reps, and some workouts entail moderate weight and moderate rep ranges.

One of the great things about undulating periodization is that it requires less organization and planning than the two other methods. For instance, if one day you feel tired or sick, you can reduce weight and increase reps. On the flip side, if you feel extra motivated and strong one day, you can go very heavy. And while it may seem as though a less structured training system would be less effective than a highly regimented one, research has found that undulating periodized programs are just as effective as linear models at developing strength, power, and muscle mass. This is likely due to the sporadic nature of the program. In the undulating model, the different types of strength training (heavy, moderate, light) are cycled repeatedly from day to day, which helps to keep the muscles from getting used to the stimulus.

The following undulating plan is perfect for turning lagging limbs into lean, muscular arms. You'll train arms twice per week with different weight and reps each time. Simply add Workout 1 to your first workout of the week and Workout 2 to any workout that's at least two days later.

4-WEEK UNDULATING PERIODIZATION FOR ARMS

WEEKS 1 & 2

EXERCISE	SETS/REPS	REST
WEEK 1: WORKOUT 1		
Barbell Curl	3/4–6	3 min.
Preacher Curl	3/4–6	3 min.
Incline Dumbbell Curl	3/4–6	3 min.
Triceps Pressdown	3/4–6	3 min.
Lying Triceps Extension	3/4–6	3 min.
Dumbbell Overhead Extension	3/4–6	3 min.
WORKOUT 2		
Close-grip Bench Press	3/16–20	
SUPERSET WITH		
Seated Dumbbell Alternating Curl	3/16–20	1–2 min.
Cable Overhead Extension	3/16–20	
SUPERSET WITH		
Cable High Curl	3/16–20	1–2 min.
Rope Triceps Pressdown		
SUPERSET WITH		
Rope Hammer Curl	3/16–20	
	3/16–20	1–2 min.

EXERCISE	SETS/REPS	REST
WEEK 2: WORKOUT 1		
EZ-bar Curl	3/7–10	2 min.
Behind-the-back Cable Curl	3/7–10	2 min.
Dumbbell Concentration Curl	3/7–10	2 min.
Close-grip Bench Press	3/7–10	2 min.
Machine Tricep Extension	3/7–10	2 min.
Reverse-grip Triceps Pressdown	3/7–10	2 min.
WORKOUT 2		
Barbell Curl	3/11–15	
SUPERSET WITH		
Lying Triceps Extension	3/11–15	1–2 min.
Supine Incline Dumbbell Curl	3/11–15	
SUPERSET WITH		
Incline Lying Triceps Extension	3/11–15	1–2 min.
Cable Curl	3/11–15	
SUPERSET WITH		
Triceps Pressdown	3/11–15	1–2 min.

WEEKS 3 & 4

EXERCISE	SETS/REPS	REST
WEEK 3: WORKOUT 1		
Barbell Curl	3/16–20	1 min.
Preacher Curl	3/16–20	1 min.
Incline Dumbbell Curl	3/16–20	1 min.
Triceps Pressdown	3/16–20	1 min.
Lying Triceps Extension	3/16–20	1 min.
Dumbbell Overhead Extension	3/16–20	1 min.

EXERCISE	SETS/REPS	REST
WORKOUT 2		
Close-grip Bench Press	3/7–10	
SUPERSET WITH		
Seated Dumbbell Alternating Curl	3/7–10	2 min.
Cable Overhead Extension	3/7–10	
SUPERSET WITH		
Cable High Curl	3/7–20	2 min.
Rope Triceps Pressdown	3/7–10	
SUPERSET WITH		
Rope Hammer Curl	3/7–10	2 min.

EXERCISE	SETS/REPS	REST
WEEK 4: WORKOUT 1		
EZ-bar Curl	3/11–15	1–2 min.
Behind-the-back Cable Curl	3/11–15	1–2 min.
Dumbbell Concentration Curl	3/11–15	1–2 min.
Close-grip Bench Press	3/11–15	1–2 min.
Machine Triceps Extension	3/11–15	1–2 min.
Reverse-grip Triceps Pressdown	3/11–15	1–2 min.
WORKOUT 2		
Barbell Curl	3/4–6	
SUPERSET WITH		
Lying Triceps Extension	3/4–6	2–3 min.
Supine Incline Dumbbell Curl	3/4–6	
SUPERSET WITH		
Incline Lying Triceps Extension	3/4–6	2–3 min.
Cable Curl	3/4–6	
SUPERSET WITH		
Triceps Pressdown	3/4–6	2–3 min.

CHAPTER 4

Lift TO Burn

Blast body fat by hitting the weights with these tried-and-true principles and workouts

"**I** need to lose weight, so I'm just going to go on a diet."

"I need to lose weight, so I'm just going to do cardio."

There are a couple of fundamental problems with making one or both of the above statements. First, you should be clear on what kind of weight you want to lose. You want to lose body fat, period. Losing muscle is never a good thing, as it will slow your metabolism and actually decrease fat burning. Second, there's no mention of lifting weights. Too many women (and men, for that matter) shun the weights when their goal is to drop pounds and lean out, but in doing so they've eliminated one of the best ways to achieve their objective. When it comes to burning body fat, diet and cardio are critical for success. Yet how you train with the iron can also have a huge impact on the amount of body fat you drop. Hit the weights hard—and wisely—and your body will shed excess blubber faster than ever.

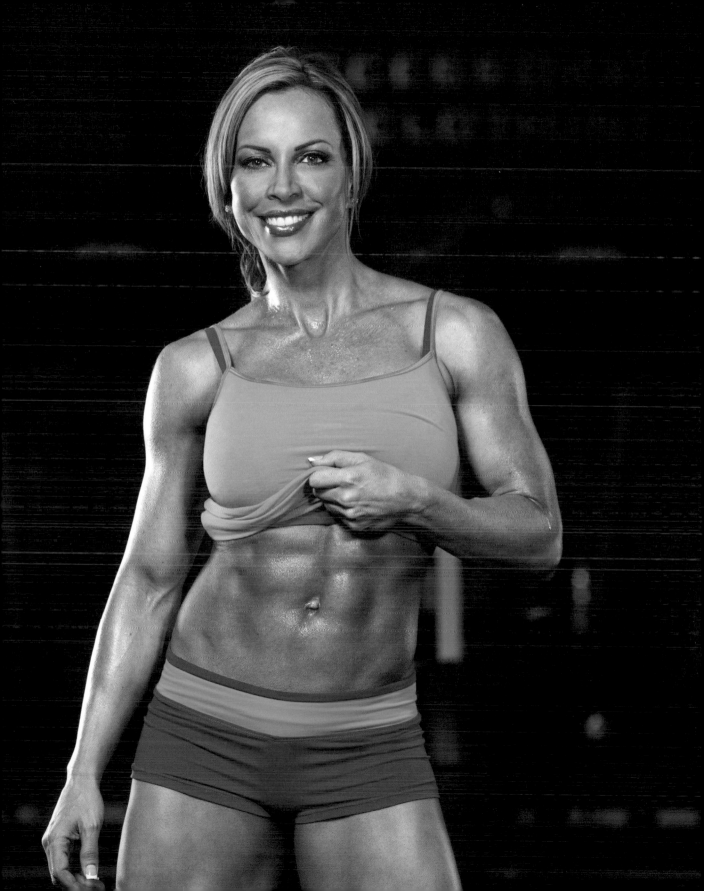

The
FAT-BURNING
FOUR

There are four training variables you can manipulate to increase the amount of fat you burn through lifting weights. If you control these variables properly, you can create a weight-training program that simultaneously melts fat while building lean muscle and strength.

1

EXERCISE SELECTION

First, consider the exercises you use. Research suggests that using free-weight, multijoint exercises such as the squat, bench press, shoulder press, and bentover row maximizes the number of calories burned compared with machine exercises or single-joint isolation moves. This is likely due to the fact that multijoint exercises utilize more muscle groups to help the target muscles lift the weight. In fact, one study found that when subjects did barbell squats, they burned 50% more calories than by doing leg presses. For this reason, we've included several free-weight, multijoint exercises in the workout.

2

WEIGHT, REP COUNT

Another variable to consider is the amount of weight you use. Doing high reps with light weight will burn more calories during the workout. College of New Jersey researchers found that when subjects used a weight that allowed them to complete 10 reps on the bench press, they burned about 10% more calories than when they used a weight that limited them to five reps. The more reps you do, the more calories you burn.

On the flip side, research suggests that although using heavier weight for fewer reps burns fewer calories during the workout, it burns more calories after the workout. Studies have shown that when you train with heavy weights that limit you to six reps per set, the boost in your metabolic rate over two days is more than double what you get when using light weights that allow you to complete 12 reps per set.

So what do you do: lift heavy or go light? We suggest you do both. This program uses heavy weight for fewer reps on some exercises and very light weight for very high reps on others to provide the best of both worlds. You'll be a calorie-burning machine both during and after your workout.

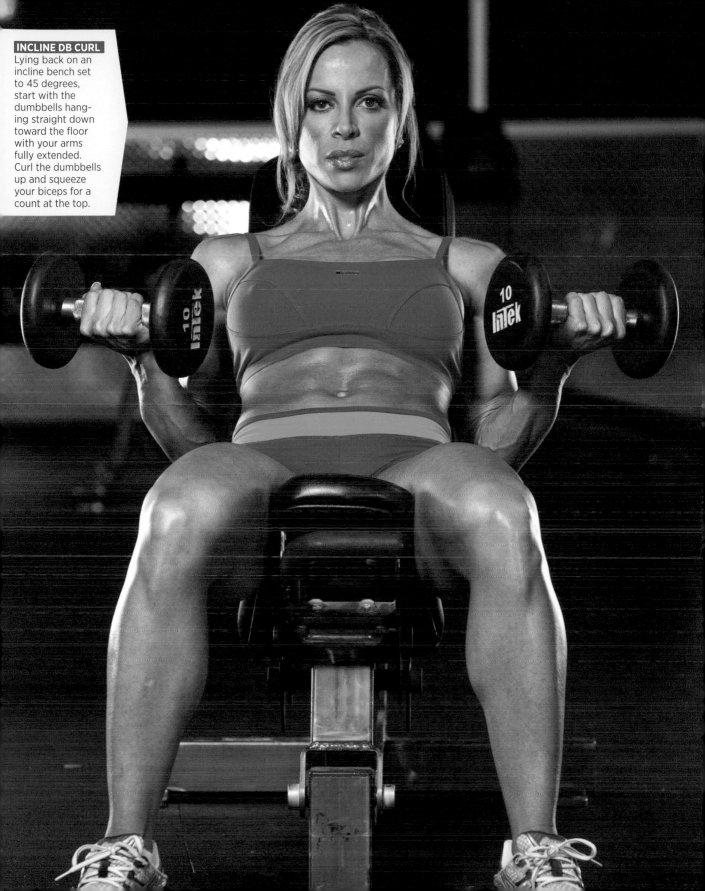

INCLINE DB CURL
Lying back on an incline bench set to 45 degrees, start with the dumbbells hanging straight down toward the floor with your arms fully extended. Curl the dumbbells up and squeeze your biceps for a count at the top.

3

REP SPEED

Research has shown that doing reps in a fast, explosive manner can increase the number of calories you burn by more than 10% as compared to doing reps in a slow, controlled manner. Plus, the fast-rep exercises resulted in a bigger boost in metabolic rate after the workout was over. And of course, boosting metabolism means burning more calories and fat at rest. This is why you'll start each major muscle group with explosive-rep training (such as power pushups for chest) in the Lift to Burn program.

Explosive-rep training is to be treated differently than your typical sets. Normally, you'll select as much weight as you can handle for a given rep count and reach failure during the set or come close to it. When performing explosive reps, you will neither use heavy weight nor train to failure, for two simple reasons:

(1) You don't want to injure yourself, and

(2) the whole point of training explosively is to do every rep as fast as possible; also, when the weight is heavy and/or you get close to reaching failure, rep speed slows down considerably, which defeats the purpose.

When doing explosive-rep sets, select a weight that allows you to complete about 25 reps, but keep your rep counts low, like you'll see in this program, with sets of 5–8. The weight will feel very light, you won't reach failure, and you'll feel like you can keep going, but stop the set anyway. You'll have plenty of opportunities to reach failure on subsequent exercises.

POWER PUSHUP
Explode out of the bottom of the pushup so that your hands leave the floor each rep. Advanced trainees can clap at the top. Land on soft elbows (not locked out).

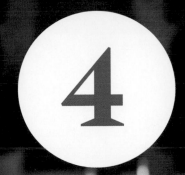

REST PERIODS

The fourth variable to consider is the rest period you allow yourself between sets. Research has shown that if you cut your rest periods down from three minutes to just 30 seconds, you can increase the number of calories you burn during the workout by more than 50%. These shorter rest periods also lead to a greater increase in the metabolic boost that follows the workout.

One way to ensure your breaks stay brief is to use supersets, the widely used training technique of doing two exercises back-to-back without resting. Researchers from Syracuse University had subjects perform a chest, back, biceps, triceps, quads, and hamstrings workout that consisted of either supersets, or straight sets with one minute of rest between sets. They reported that when the subjects did the superset workout, they burned 35% more calories per minute during the training session and burned 35% more total calories during the hour after the workout was over. In our program, you'll use supersets for each major muscle group. You'll also rest just 30 seconds between straight sets that involve light weight.

Lift to Burn Training Program

OVERVIEW

>**Workouts per week:** *4*
(To be done on whatever days you prefer)
>**Number of times each body part is trained weekly:**
Once, with the exception of abs (twice)
>**Volume per body part per week:**
10–13 sets for larger body parts; 6–10 for smaller body parts
>**Rest periods between sets:**
From 30 seconds to 2 minutes
>**Intensity-boosting techniques employed:**
Explosive-rep training, supersets

>*In addition to lifting workouts, do 3–4 steady-state cardio workouts per week. When doing cardio on lifting days, either do it in the morning in a separate session from or after lifting if you're doing both in the same workout.*

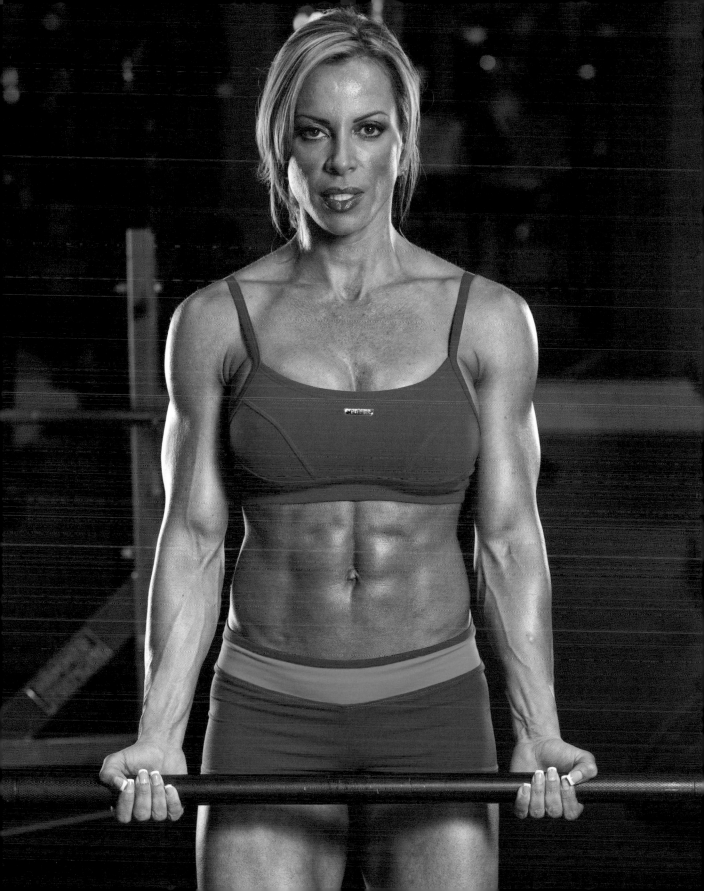

DUMBBELL POWER ROW
Perform a one-arm dumbbell row more explosively than normal, and turn your working-side shoulder up at the top of the rep so the dumbbell can travel past your chest. Then control the dumbbell's descent.

Workout 1 – Chest, Triceps

MUSCLE GROUP	EXERCISE	SETS/REPS	REST
Chest			
	Power Pushup	2/5–8	30 sec.
	Bench Press	2/6–8	1–2 min.
	Incline Dumbbell Press	3/6–8	-
	SUPERSET WITH		
	Incline Dumbbell Flye	3/20	1 min.
Triceps			
	Smith Machine Close-grip Bench Press Throw	2/5–8	30 sec.
	Lying Triceps Extension	3/20	-
	SUPERSET WITH		
	Triceps Pressdown	3/20	30 sec.

Workout 2 – Legs

MUSCLE GROUP	EXERCISE	SETS/REPS	REST
Quads/Glutes			
	Jump Squat	2/3–5	30 sec.
	Leg Press	3/20	30 sec.
Quads			
	Leg Extension	3/25	-
	SUPERSET WITH		
Hamstrings			
	Leg Curl	3/25	30 sec.
	Romanian Deadlift	3/25	30 sec.
Calves			
	Standing Calf Raise	3/10	-
	SUPERSET WITH		
	Seated Calf Raise	3/30	30 sec.

Workout 3 – Shoulders

MUSCLE GROUP	EXERCISE	SETS/REPS	REST
Shoulders			
	Smith Machine Overhead Press Throw	2–3/5	30 sec.
	Barbell Upright Row	3/6–8	-
	SUPERSET WITH		
	Dumbbell Lateral Raise	3/20	1 min.
	Dumbbell Bentover Lateral Raise	3/25	30 sec.

Workout 4 – Back, Biceps

MUSCLE GROUP	EXERCISE	SETS/REPS	REST
Back			
	Dumbbell Power Row	2/8	30 sec.
	Barbell Bentover Row	2/6–8	1–2 min.
	Lat Pulldown	3/6–8	-
	SUPERSET WITH		
	Straight-arm Pulldown	3/20	1 min.
Biceps			
	Smith Machine Curl Throw	2/8	30 sec.
	Incline Dumbbell Curl	3/20	-
	SUPERSET WITH		
	Prone Incline Dumbbell Curl	3/20	30 sec.

Six-Pack Sizzle

We recommend training abs twice a week on the Lift to Burn program—after legs in Workout 2 and after shoulders in Workout 3. In Workout 2, you'll superset two exercises to burn more calories both during and after the workout. In Workout 3, you'll do straight sets with additional weight to increase post-workout fat-burning.

Workout 2 (after legs)

EXERCISE	SETS/REPS	REST
Hip Thrust	3/To failure	-
SUPERSET WITH		
Crossover Crunch	3/To failure	30 sec.

Workout 3 (after shoulders)

EXERCISE	SETS/REPS	REST
Cable Crunch	3/10	30 sec.
Oblique Cable Crunch	3/20	-

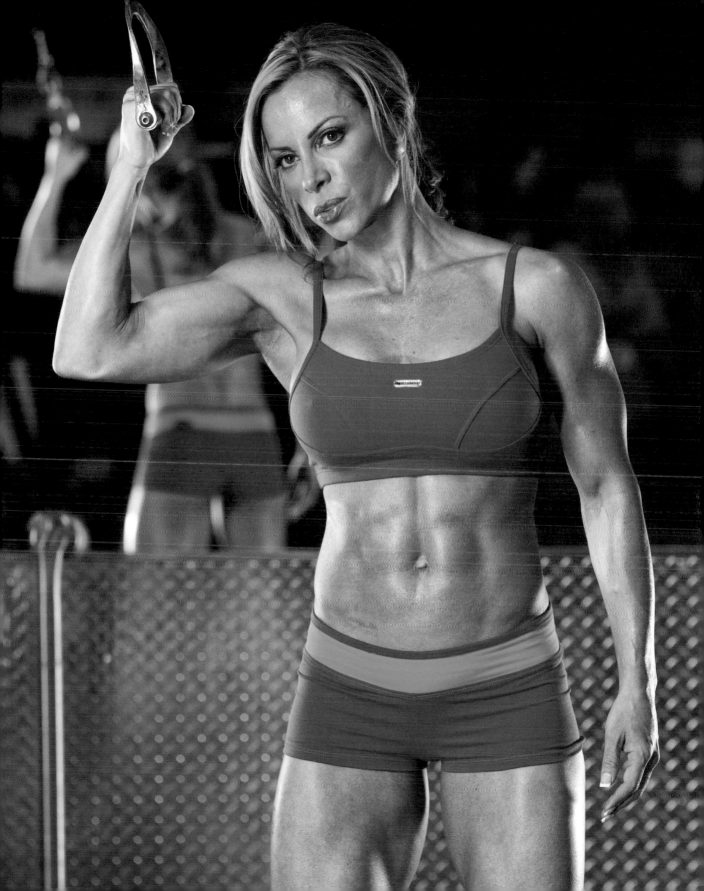

CHAPTER 5

Combo It

Pressed for time and trying to get the most burn for your buck? Give combination exercises a try.

I t's your lunch break, and you're headed to the gym. On the way over, you're planning the workout: Two body parts in about 45 minutes. If that machine isn't available, do this exercise instead...

By the time you walk through the door, you have it all figured out—complete with backup plans. If there's one thing women are truly great at, it's multitasking. That ability won't just help you plan your workout, though; it can help you get more out of it in the form of "combo exercises"—combining two or more exercises into one fluid movement. This multitasking training technique can help you burn more fat than with individual movements, help you attain functional fitness, and shake up a stale routine all at the same time.

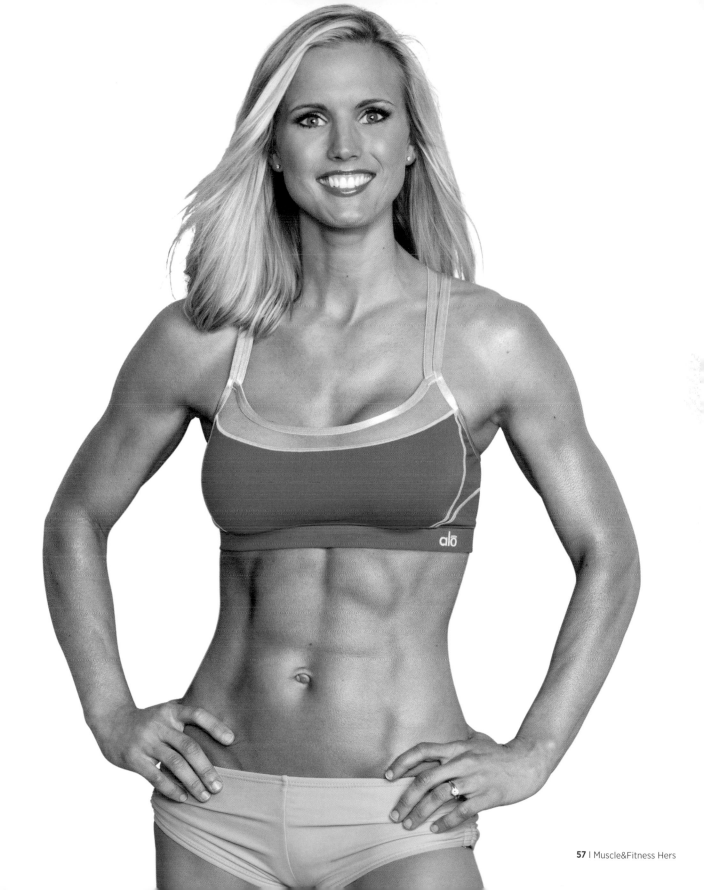

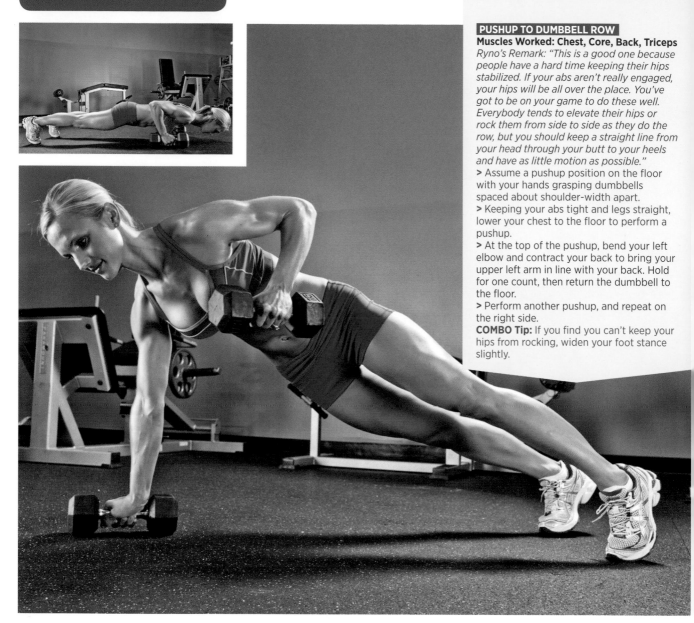

PUSHUP TO DUMBBELL ROW
Muscles Worked: Chest, Core, Back, Triceps
Ryno's Remark: "This is a good one because people have a hard time keeping their hips stabilized. If your abs aren't really engaged, your hips will be all over the place. You've got to be on your game to do these well. Everybody tends to elevate their hips or rock them from side to side as they do the row, but you should keep a straight line from your head through your butt to your heels and have as little motion as possible."
> Assume a pushup position on the floor with your hands grasping dumbbells spaced about shoulder-width apart.
> Keeping your abs tight and legs straight, lower your chest to the floor to perform a pushup.
> At the top of the pushup, bend your left elbow and contract your back to bring your upper left arm in line with your back. Hold for one count, then return the dumbbell to the floor.
> Perform another pushup, and repeat on the right side.
COMBO Tip: If you find you can't keep your hips from rocking, widen your foot stance slightly.

Five Keys to Combo Moves

1 **MORE BANG FOR YOUR BUCK**
"We weren't designed to just sit at a plate-loaded machine endlessly," says Jim Ryno, founder of LIFT personal training studios and a nationally recognized personal trainer who works with clients in New York (*jimryno.me*). "We were meant to move differently, so combination moves are more functional. Probably the single-best benefit is upping your intensity so that you can get more done in less time and increase your caloric expenditure."

2 **ENDLESS VARIETY**
Combination exercises allow you to be creative. With a little thought, almost any muscle groups can be paired together: back with arms, chest with core. Legs can easily be combined with shoulders, arms, or back—even chest, if you're willing to use a little bit of plyometrics (think burpees).

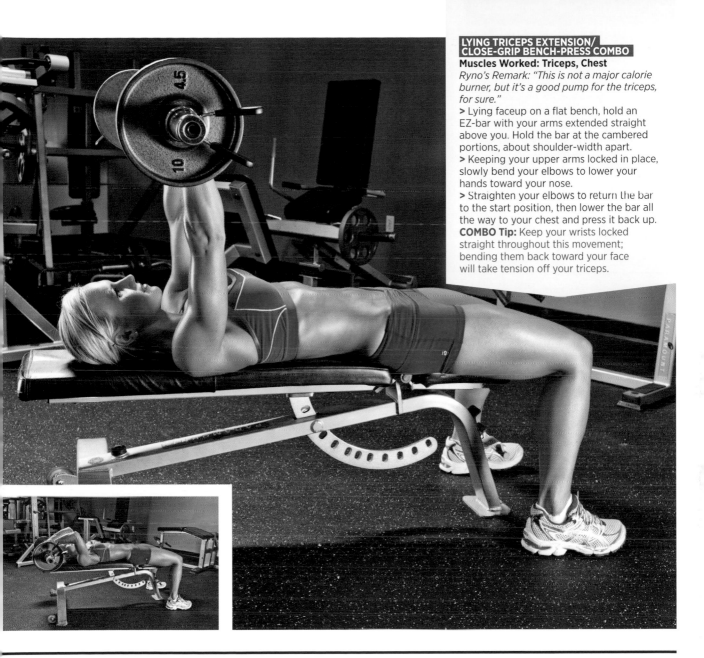

LYING TRICEPS EXTENSION/ CLOSE-GRIP BENCH-PRESS COMBO

Muscles Worked: Triceps, Chest

Ryno's Remark: "This is not a major calorie burner, but it's a good pump for the triceps, for sure."

> Lying faceup on a flat bench, hold an EZ-bar with your arms extended straight above you. Hold the bar at the cambered portions, about shoulder-width apart.

> Keeping your upper arms locked in place, slowly bend your elbows to lower your hands toward your nose.

> Straighten your elbows to return the bar to the start position, then lower the bar all the way to your chest and press it back up.

COMBO Tip: Keep your wrists locked straight throughout this movement; bending them back toward your face will take tension off your triceps.

3 TREAD LIGHTLY

"Combo exercises aren't necessarily for newbies," Ryno warns. "Before you start implementing them, you should have a solid foundation built through basic strength movements, because they take some coordination. Until you have that, you're not going to benefit 100%." Another time to avoid combo moves is when you're trying to build size; that extra calorie burn is custom-made for higher heart rates and caloric deficits.

4 CONTROL YOUR TEMPO

Avoid the temptation to rush through any segment of a combination movement. Just as when performing single-joint exercises, an even tempo will help you get the most out of the movement. "Form is key," Ryno says. "You have to slow down and visualize working each muscle."

5 PROGRAM OVERHAUL NOT NECESSARY

You don't have to go through an entire workout of combination moves to reap their benefits; just sprinkle one or two into a session when you're trying to lean out, looking for a new challenge, and/ or wanting to break through a training plateau. Get lean and have fun—simultaneously.

Combo Routines

You don't have to drastically change your program to start using combo moves. Any day you're short on time and are looking for an intense full-body workout, try one of these sample routines.

Workout 1
STRAIGHT-UP COMBO

Do four straight sets of each exercise for 15–20 reps each; on the last set perform a dropset by reducing the weight by 20%–30% and continuing. Rest one minute between all sets and exercises.
• *Squat Jump/Pullup with Muscle-Up*
• *Exercise Ball Pike-Up with Inverted Pushup*
• *Dumbbell Lunge/Curl/Overhead Press Combo*
• *Lying Triceps Extension/Close-Grip Bench-Press Combo*

Workout 2
COMBO CIRCUITS

Do one set of 15–20 reps for each exercise and then move immediately to the next exercise, resting only as long as it takes you to set up the weights. Once you have completed all five exercises, rest one minute. Complete this circuit four times.
• *Dumbbell Squat to Push-Press*
• *Pushup to Dumbbell Row*
• *Burpees (not pictured)*
• *Lying Triceps Extension/Close-Grip Bench-Press Combo*
• *Dumbbell Lunge/Curl/Overhead-Press Combo*

Workout 3
ACCELERATED COMBOS

Do three sets of 15–20 reps for each exercise, but instead of resting between sets do jumping jacks for one minute and then move immediately into the next set.
• *Exercise Ball Pike-Up with Inverted Pushup*
• *Pushup to Dumbbell Row*
• *Lying Triceps Extension/Close-Grip Bench-Press Combo*
• *Squat Jump/Pullup with Muscle-Up*
• *Dumbbell Squat to Push-Press*
• *Dumbbell Lunge/Curl/Overhead-Press Combo*

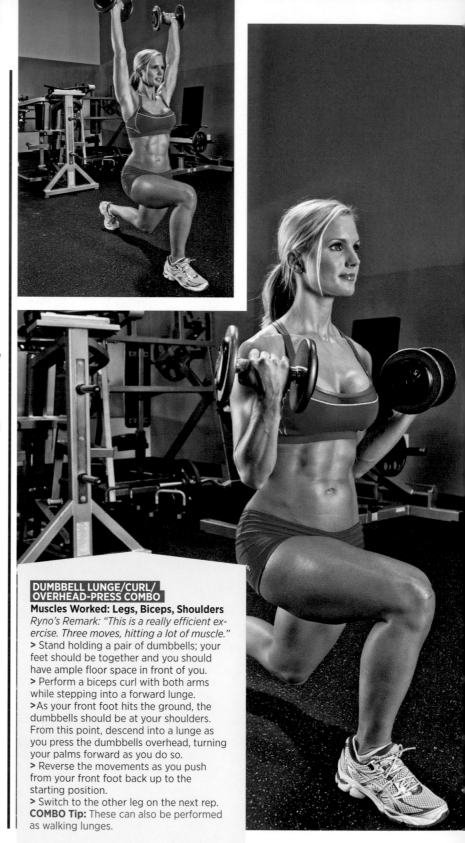

DUMBBELL LUNGE/CURL/ OVERHEAD-PRESS COMBO
Muscles Worked: Legs, Biceps, Shoulders
Ryno's Remark: "This is a really efficient exercise. Three moves, hitting a lot of muscle."
> Stand holding a pair of dumbbells; your feet should be together and you should have ample floor space in front of you.
> Perform a biceps curl with both arms while stepping into a forward lunge.
>As your front foot hits the ground, the dumbbells should be at your shoulders. From this point, descend into a lunge as you press the dumbbells overhead, turning your palms forward as you do so.
> Reverse the movements as you push from your front foot back up to the starting position.
> Switch to the other leg on the next rep.
COMBO Tip: These can also be performed as walking lunges.

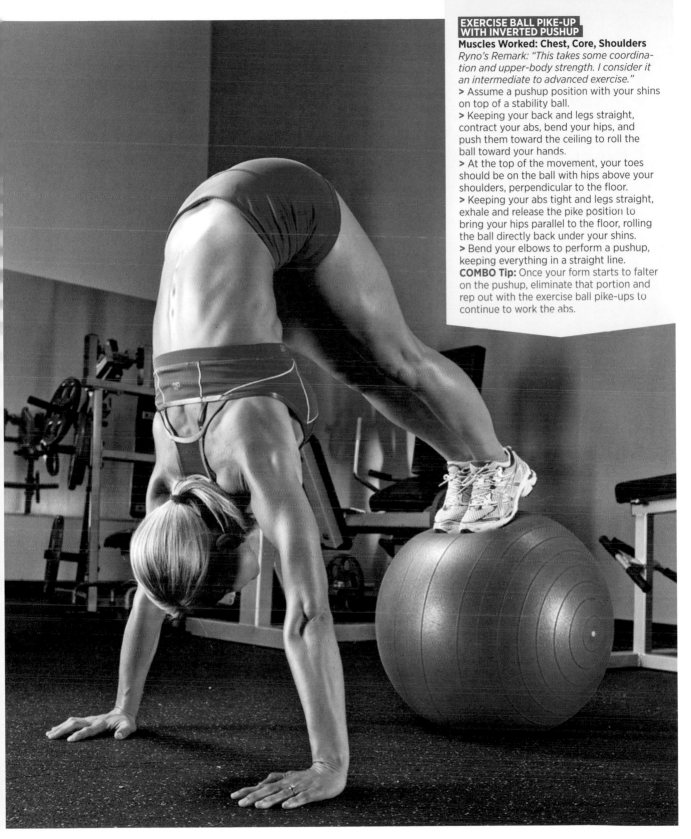

EXERCISE BALL PIKE-UP WITH INVERTED PUSHUP

Muscles Worked: Chest, Core, Shoulders

Ryno's Remark: "This takes some coordination and upper-body strength. I consider it an intermediate to advanced exercise."

> Assume a pushup position with your shins on top of a stability ball.

> Keeping your back and legs straight, contract your abs, bend your hips, and push them toward the ceiling to roll the ball toward your hands.

> At the top of the movement, your toes should be on the ball with hips above your shoulders, perpendicular to the floor.

> Keeping your abs tight and legs straight, exhale and release the pike position to bring your hips parallel to the floor, rolling the ball directly back under your shins.

> Bend your elbows to perform a pushup, keeping everything in a straight line.

COMBO Tip: Once your form starts to falter on the pushup, eliminate that portion and rep out with the exercise ball pike-ups to continue to work the abs.

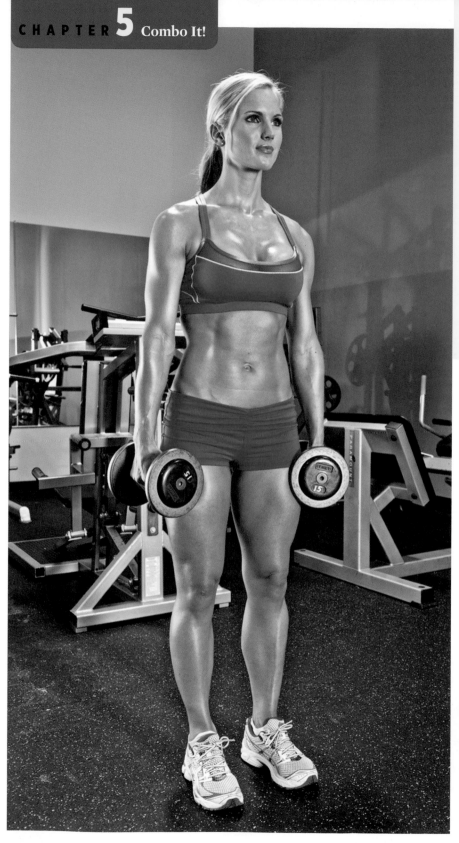

DUMBBELL SQUAT TO PUSH-PRESS
Muscles Worked: Legs, Core, Shoulders

Ryno's Remark: "This doesn't take a ton of coordination if you're good at squats. If your abs are engaged and your hips are pushed back, you can handle a good amount of weight. You're not just relying on the shoulders on the press—you're getting some energy from the ground on your squat. You're explosive on the way up and the way down."

> Stand with your feet shoulder-width apart, holding a pair of dumbbells at your shoulders, palms facing in.
> Push your hips back until you reach about 90 degrees of flexion in the knees; your quads should be parallel to the floor.
> Keeping your abs tight and, while looking straight ahead, press forcefully out of the squat while simultaneously pressing the dumbbells—and turning your palms forward—overhead.
> Lower the dumbbells to your shoulders as you sink back into a squat.

COMBO Tip: Use a light pair of dumbbells until you learn to feel the movement correctly, then add weight.

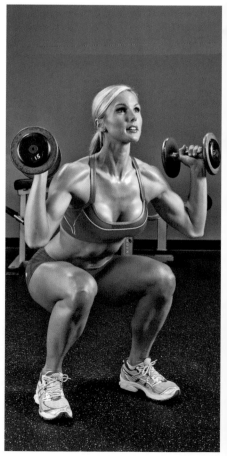

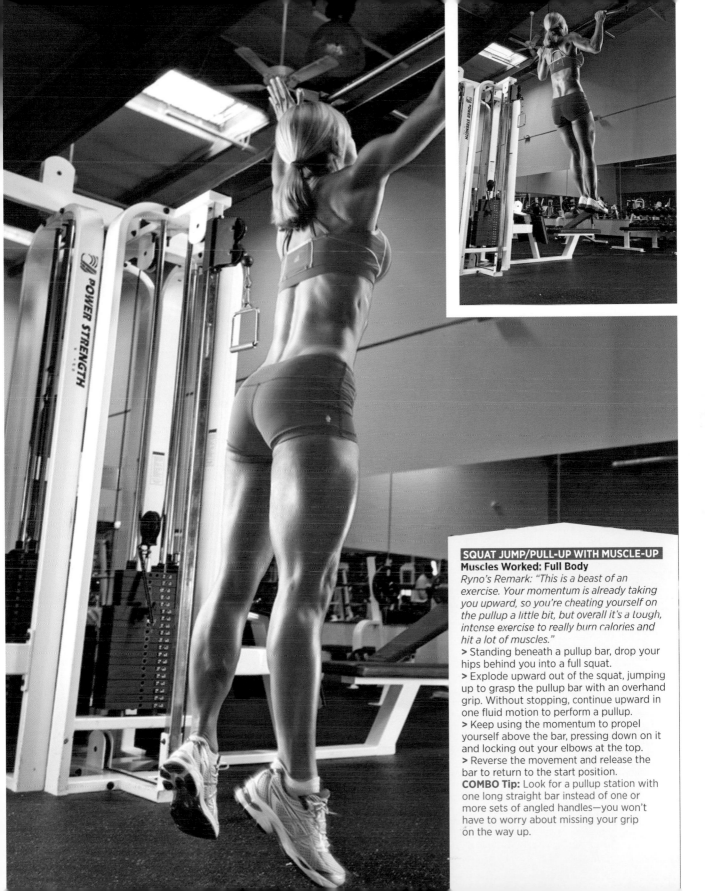

SQUAT JUMP/PULL-UP WITH MUSCLE-UP
Muscles Worked: Full Body

Ryno's Remark: "This is a beast of an exercise. Your momentum is already taking you upward, so you're cheating yourself on the pullup a little bit, but overall it's a tough, intense exercise to really burn calories and hit a lot of muscles."

> Standing beneath a pullup bar, drop your hips behind you into a full squat.
> Explode upward out of the squat, jumping up to grasp the pullup bar with an overhand grip. Without stopping, continue upward in one fluid motion to perform a pullup.
> Keep using the momentum to propel yourself above the bar, pressing down on it and locking out your elbows at the top.
> Reverse the movement and release the bar to return to the start position.

COMBO Tip: Look for a pullup station with one long straight bar instead of one or more sets of angled handles—you won't have to worry about missing your grip on the way up.

Tabata Time

Burn fat, build muscle, get stronger. We've got your all-in-one solution: Tabata interval training

We all want results, and the faster and easier we can get 'em, the better. Yet for decades the mainstream media have preached the gospel of the fat-burning zone, an outdated mindset that says if you want to burn fat, you should perform cardio at a low-intensity aerobic pace for

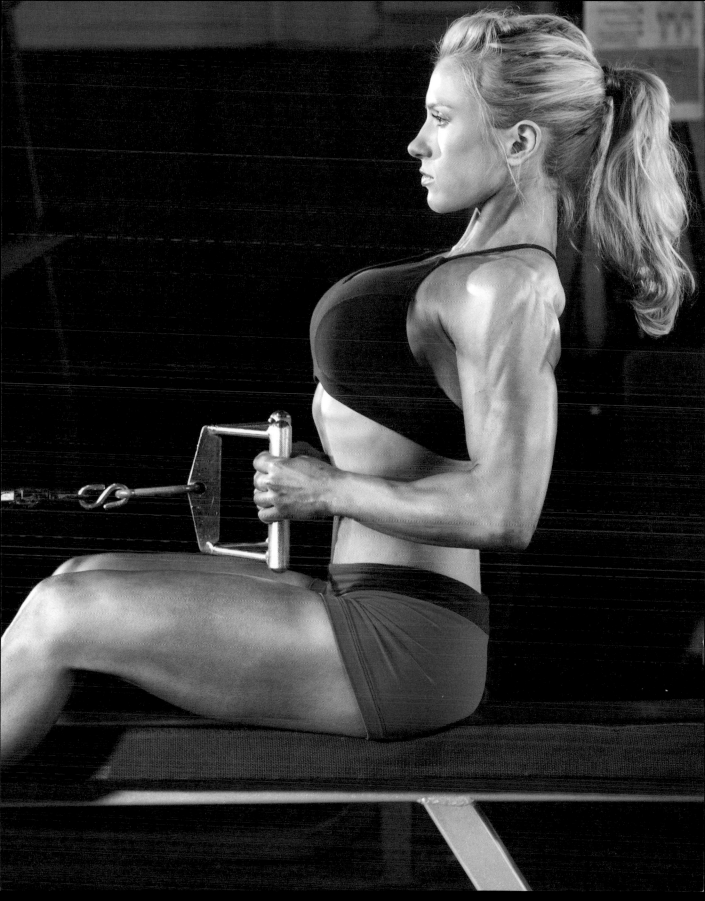

What Is

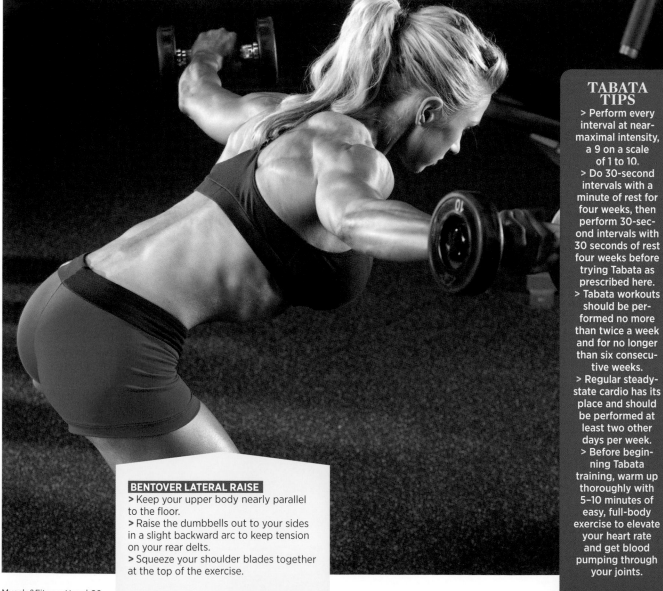

TABATA TIPS

> Perform every interval at near-maximal intensity, a 9 on a scale of 1 to 10.
> Do 30-second intervals with a minute of rest for four weeks, then perform 30-second intervals with 30 seconds of rest four weeks before trying Tabata as prescribed here.
> Tabata workouts should be performed no more than twice a week and for no longer than six consecutive weeks.
> Regular steady-state cardio has its place and should be performed at least two other days per week.
> Before beginning Tabata training, warm up thoroughly with 5–10 minutes of easy, full-body exercise to elevate your heart rate and get blood pumping through your joints.

BENTOVER LATERAL RAISE
> Keep your upper body nearly parallel to the floor.
> Raise the dumbbells out to your sides in a slight backward arc to keep tension on your rear delts.
> Squeeze your shoulder blades together at the top of the exercise.

Tabata?

Tabata is a form of interval training in which you exercise intensely for 20 seconds and rest for 10 seconds. You perform eight cycles, or sets, of this 20:10 work:rest ratio, so each exercise or cardio interval takes four minutes to complete. The training protocol was designed by Izumi Tabata, Ph.D., to better train Japanese speed skaters. He discovered that when athletes performed eight cycles of 20:10 intervals, they increased both their aerobic (endurance) capacity and their anaerobic (short bursts of work) capacity more than when they did moderate-intensity cardio.

Three Reasons to Try Tabata

1

BURNS MORE FAT.
Studies show that high-intensity interval training like Tabata burns fat more effectively than slow, steady cardio sessions.

2

MAKES YOU STRONGER.
Tabata training enhances explosive energy, which can help you complete more reps with a given weight or use more weight to finish a given number of reps.

3

HELPS BUILD LEAN MUSCLE.
High reps and little rest between sets increase the amount of blood vessels feeding your muscles, which can lead to more energy during workouts, along with better recovery and progress afterward.

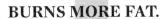

Getting Started

We recommend the following Tabata workouts depending on your level of experience:

Beginner
Two four-minute sessions with two minutes of rest in between

Intermediate
Two four-minute sessions with one minute of rest in between

Advanced
Four four-minute sessions with one minute of rest in between

SHOULDERS

EXERCISE	SETS/TIME	REST
Standing Overhead Press	8/20 sec.	10 sec.
Lateral Raise	8/20 sec.	10 sec.
Bentover Lateral Raise	8/20 sec.	10 sec.

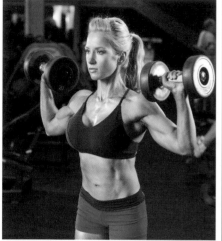

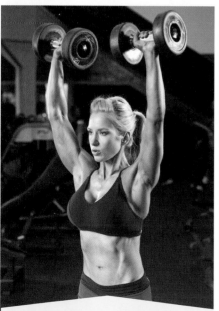

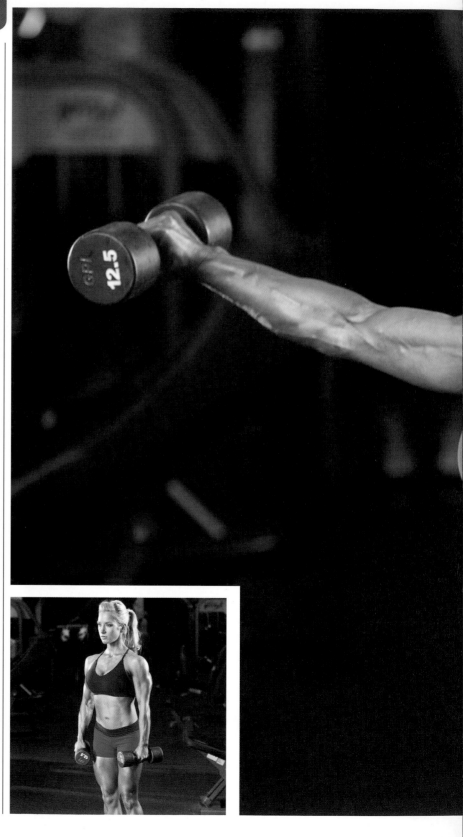

STANDING OVERHEAD PRESS
> Keep a slight arch in your lower back and your core tight throughout the exercise.
> Press the dumbbells in a slight arc from your shoulders to overhead.
> Avoid locking out your elbows at the top, to keep continuous tension on your delts.

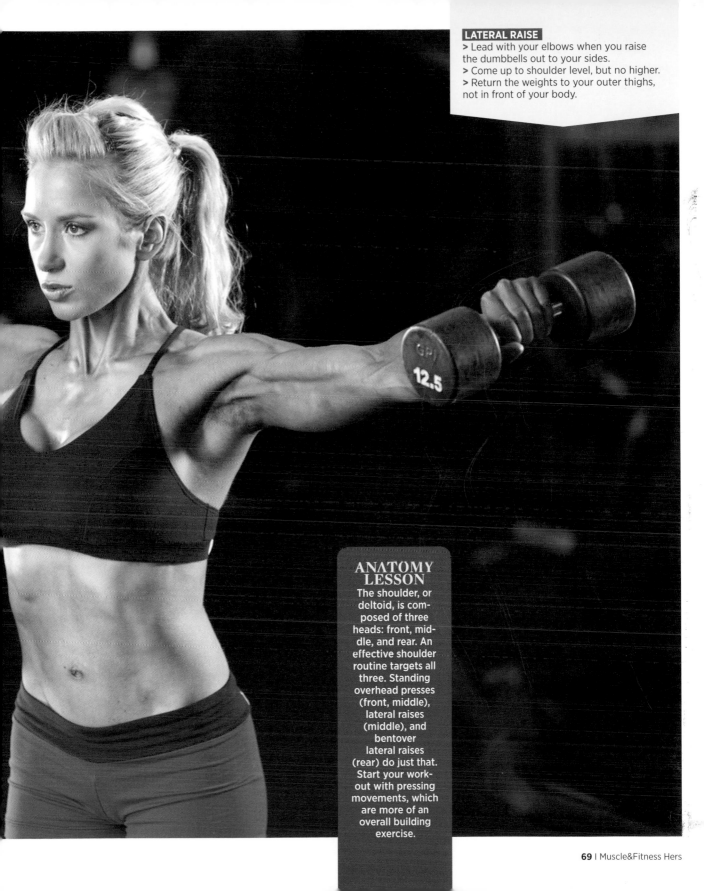

LATERAL RAISE
> Lead with your elbows when you raise the dumbbells out to your sides.
> Come up to shoulder level, but no higher.
> Return the weights to your outer thighs, not in front of your body.

ANATOMY LESSON
The shoulder, or deltoid, is composed of three heads: front, middle, and rear. An effective shoulder routine targets all three. Standing overhead presses (front, middle), lateral raises (middle), and bentover lateral raises (rear) do just that. Start your workout with pressing movements, which are more of an overall building exercise.

LEGS

EXERCISE	SETS/TIME	REST
Body-weight Squat	8/20 sec.	10 sec.
Leg Extension	8/20 sec.	10 sec.
Lying Leg Curl	8/20 sec.	10 sec.

ANATOMY LESSON

The legs are composed of the quads on the front of the thigh, and the hamstrings and glutes on the back. An effective leg workout typically starts with a multijoint exercise like the squat that hits all three areas. Follow up with isolation moves that target the quads (leg extension) and hams (lying leg curl) separately.

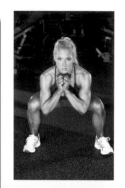

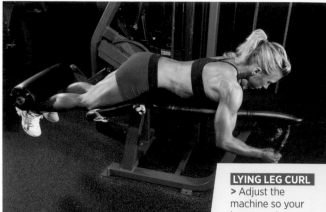

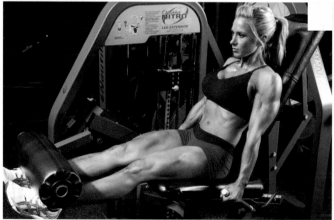

LYING LEG CURL
> Adjust the machine so your knees are just past the edge of the bench.
> Set the padded bar just above your heels.
> Keep a slight bend in your knees at the bottom of the exercise to keep tension on your hamstrings.

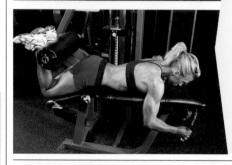

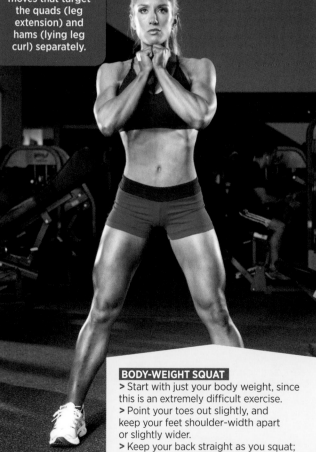

BODY-WEIGHT SQUAT
> Start with just your body weight, since this is an extremely difficult exercise.
> Point your toes out slightly, and keep your feet shoulder-width apart or slightly wider.
> Keep your back straight as you squat; don't lean over your knees.

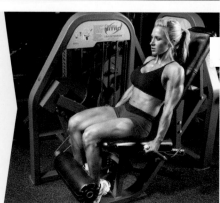

LEG EXTENSION
> Adjust the machine so the backs of your knees are flush with the edge of the seat.
> Keep your back flat against the backpad and set the padded bar at your lower ankles.
> Squeeze your quads at the top of the movement.

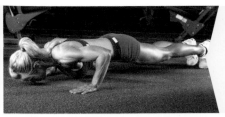

PUSHUP
(Chest, triceps, front delts)
> Keep your back flat and don't let your hips sag.
> Avoid locking out your elbows, to keep tension on your chest and triceps.
> Perform on your knees if you fatigue early.

MUSCLE-BUILDING

EXERCISE	SETS/TIME	REST
Pushup	8/20 sec.	10 sec.
Bentover Dumbbell Row	8/20 sec.	10 sec.
Dumbbell Lunge	8/20 sec.	10 sec.
Crunch	8/20 sec.	10 sec.

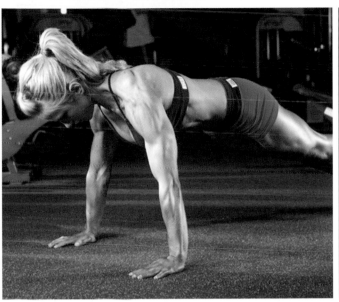

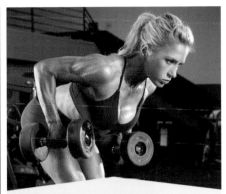

BENTOVER DUMBBELL ROW
(Back, biceps, rear delts)
> Keep your back slightly arched and your head in line with your spine.
> Pull the weights toward your hips.
> Try to squeeze your elbows together at the top of the movement.

CRUNCH TIME
In a recent study, researchers tested the muscle activity of subjects' rectus abdominis, external and internal obliques, and spinal erectors as they performed crunches at rep speeds of four seconds, two seconds, 1.5 seconds, one second, or as fast as possible. As rep speed increased, so did the activity of all four muscles. The greatest boost in muscle activity occurred in the external obliques, which were hardly involved in the crunch at slower speeds but whose activity increased by more than six times at the fastest speed. Fast reps recruit more muscle fibers in the midsection and can help turn an ab exercise like the crunch into a fairly effective oblique move.

CRUNCH
(Abs)
> Bend your knees 90 degrees, feet flat on the floor.
> Don't pull on your neck; squeeze your abs to bring your shoulders toward your thighs.
> Keep your core tight as you lower back down.

CHAPTER 7

Clear As a Bell

It's official: Kettlebells are more than a passing craze. Take advantage of this old-school training tool for a brand-new, athletically streamlined body.

The fitness industry has survived more than its fair share of fads. And we're not just talking about cringe-worthy fashion train wrecks like G-string leotards, neon spandex, and off-the-shoulder sweatshirts.

Fads have permeated the training floor, too, as health clubs, in an effort to keep members engaged, have grasped onto everything from the Reebok slide to pole dancing to Tae Bo. (Remember that? Billy Blanks sure wishes you did.)

Thus, those of you who've seen many years worth of dewy-eyed January newbies come and go—usually by February—may have been wary when your gym started importing those round cannonball-shaped weights with the handle atop them.

Here we are, though, a few years after decidedly old-school kettle-bell training reemerged on the fitness scene, and they're still growing in popularity, dramatically making the rare leap from fad to bona-fide fitness phenomenon. One very potent reason explains why: If you're after athletic curves and a body worthy of a *Hers* cover, kettlebell training works.

Joe Chakalee, certified RKC instructor and owner of Kettlebell South Bay in Torrance, CA, has designed *Hers*-approved workouts that shape the body from your shoulders to your toes—consisting of a "beginner" session for the first six weeks of kettlebell training, and an intermediate/advanced program for those ready to move up to the next level.

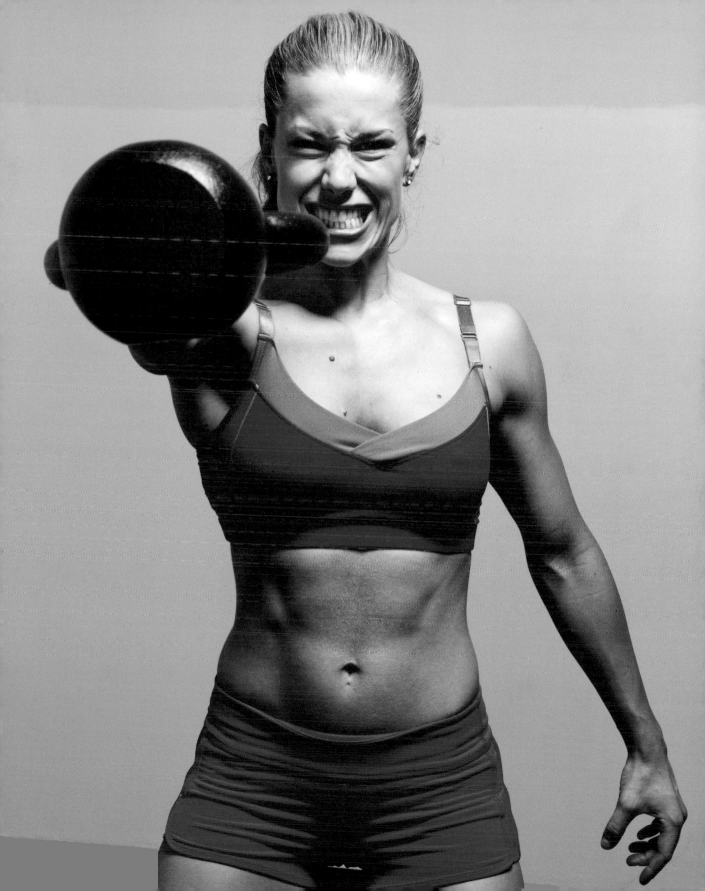

BEGINNER ROUTINE

Perform this workout up to three times
per week.

EXERCISE	SETS	REPS
Naked Turkish Get-up	3	1 per side
Two-handed Swing	10	10
Unilateral Stiff-leg Deadlift	3	5 per side
Goblet Squat	5	5
Forward Lunge	5	5 per side
Bentover Row	5	5 per side
Press	5	3 per side

Notes: Rest 45 to 90 seconds between sets, as
needed. Chakalee recommends an 18-pound
kettlebell for everything except the get-up,
which is done sans weight; once you do feel
you can handle weight on that exercise, start
with a 10-pounder.

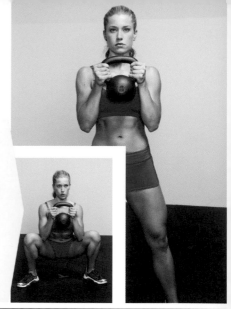

GOBLET SQUAT

GET READY: Hold the kettlebell at your
upper chest, elbows pointing down, hands
firmly holding each side of the handle. Step
into a wide sumo-style squat position.
GO: Bend at the knees and drop your torso
and butt straight down toward the floor,
as deep as you comfortably can while
keeping your feet flat on the floor. Reverse
by extending your hips and driving upward
through your heels. Maintain the natural
curve in your lower back throughout, and
keep your eyes focused forward.

TWO-HANDED SWING

GET READY: Squat down and grasp a kettlebell between your legs with both hands,
making sure to maintain the natural arch in
your lower back by tightening your core.
GO: Extend your knees and hips to generate
momentum and swing the weight in an arc
to chest level, keeping your arms extended
and your shoulders back (not allowing them
to round forward). Allow gravity to return
the kettlebell to the start position as you
bend your knees and hips.

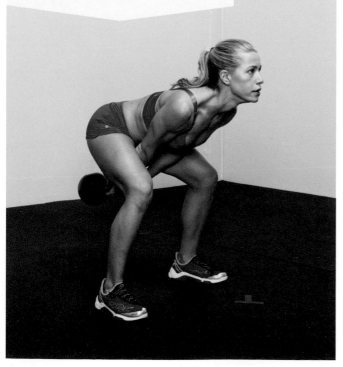

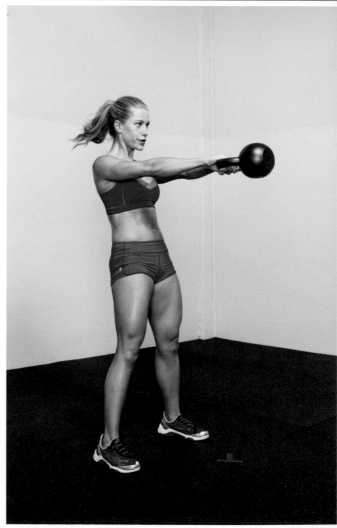

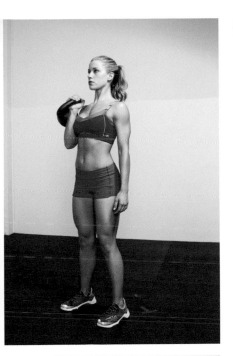

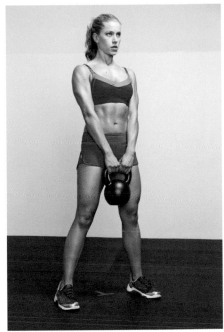

PRESS

GET READY: Clean a kettlebell to shoulder level by squatting down, grasping it between your legs with one hand, and pulling it straight up as you extend your knees and hips. As the weight reaches your waist, rotate your shoulder and bring your elbow underneath so the kettlebell is at chin level, resting against your forearm, your arm tight against your flank to help support the weight with your body (not just your wrist).

GO: Press the kettlebell powerfully overhead, rotating your wrist so your palm faces forward. Straighten your elbow; when you finish, your biceps should be near your ear. Lower it back to shoulder level and repeat for reps before setting the weight back down on the floor.

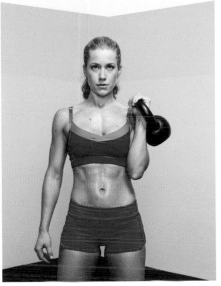

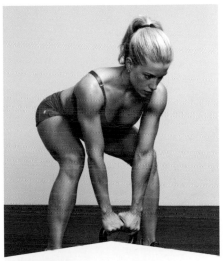

DEADLIFT

GET READY: Stand upright, feet outside shoulder width, holding a kettlebell with both hands.

GO: Keeping your back flat and head and spine aligned at all times, lean forward at the hips, leading with the weight as it lowers straight down to the floor. Stop when your upper body reaches parallel with the floor (don't let the weight touch down). From there, contract your hamstrings and glutes to return back up to an upright, standing position. Keep your feet planted firmly on the floor throughout and concentrate on not letting your lower back round as you reach the bottom position.

FORWARD LUNGE

GET READY: Holding a kettlebell in your right hand, step forward from a standing position into a lunge with your left foot.

GO: Bend both knees to lower your hips toward the floor, keeping your torso upright. Stop before your rear knee touches the floor and pass the kettlebell under your lead leg, transferring it to your left hand and returning to a standing position. Repeat, this time stepping forward with your right foot. Alternate for reps.

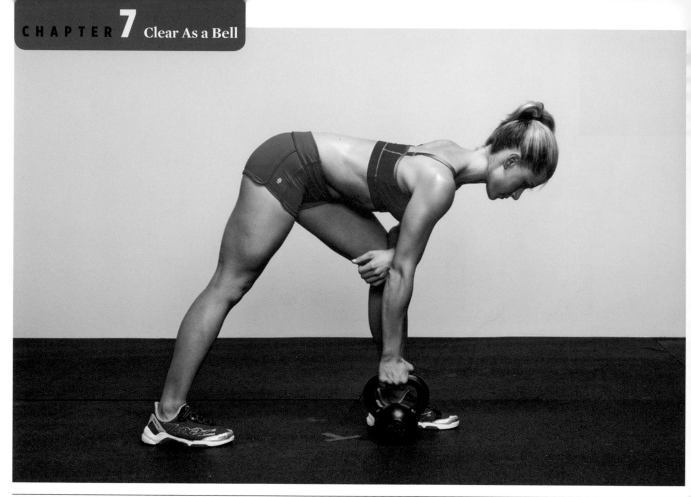

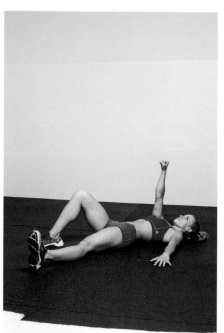

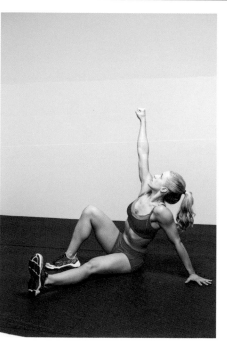

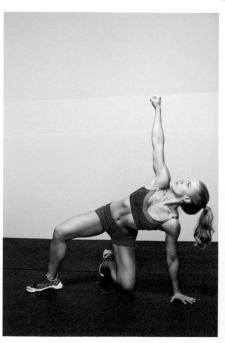

BENTOVER ROW

GET READY: Bend at your hips and hold a kettlebell with your right hand, arm hanging straight down from your shoulder girdle to the floor. Step forward with your left foot and back with your right. Place your left hand on the same-side knee for support.

GO: Pull the kettlebell toward your hip, allowing your elbow to track up toward the ceiling, keeping your lower back tight. Squeeze your shoulder blade back at the top, then lower the weight to an arm-extended position. Repeat for reps, then switch arms.

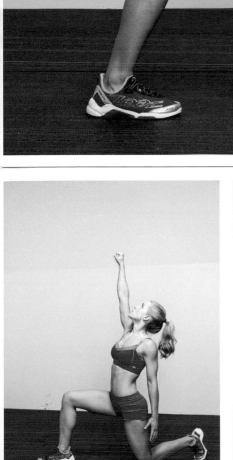

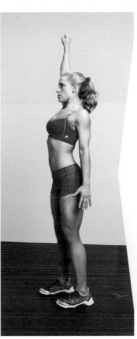

NAKED TURKISH GET-UP

GET READY: Lie faceup on the floor and hold your right hand directly above your shoulder, with your elbow and wrist locked straight, as if you were holding a kettlebell. ("Naked" means you do this exercise without the weight.)

GO: With your eyes continually on your right hand (where the weight would be), bend your right knee so your foot is flat on the floor, sit up and tilt your hips so you're supported on both feet and your left hand. Swing your left leg under your body and prop yourself up on that knee. Press through your left knee and right foot to stand upright. Follow the same pattern to return to the floor, then repeat by switching sides. That's one set.

HIGH-POWERED CALORIE BURN

Although kettlebells can seem like a masculine way to train at first blush, they are in fact extremely female-friendly, says Delaine Ross, a Russian-Kettlebell-Challenge-certified trainer based in Atlanta, GA. "Kettlebells train the body as a unit, the way we function in real life," she explains. "Isolated muscle training can bulk you up, but kettlebell-built muscles are lean and strong." Science backs Ross' enthusiastic assertions. An American Council on Exercise-sponsored study out of the University of Wisconsin-La Crosse found that kettlebell training proved to be an excellent calorie-burning activity, as subjects used an average of 272 calories over a 20-minute session of various snatches. Another study, published in the *Journal of Strength and Conditioning*, found that 10 weeks of kettlebell training translated into strength and endurance improvements in other athletic activities, augmenting the kettlebell's reputation as a universal fitness tool.

INTERMEDIATE/ADVANCED ROUTINE

Graduate to this program after at least six weeks of consistently doing the beginner program if you're new to kettlebell training. Do this program three to five times per week.

EXERCISE	SETS	REPS
Turkish Get-up	3	1 per side
Two-handed Swing	5	10
One-handed Swing	5	5 per side
Alternating Swing (switch at the top of each swing)	5	10 total
Unilateral Stiff-leg Deadlift	3	5 per side
Goblet Squat	6	5
Reverse Lunge	5	5 per side
Bentover Row	5	5 per side
Press	5	3 per side
Windmill	3	1 per side

Notes: Rest 30–60 seconds between sets, as needed. Choose either an 18-, 26-, or 31-pound kettlebell, as much as you can handle with good form, for all of the above movements except the Turkish get-up and windmill. For those two exercises, use a 10-, 14-, or 18-pound kettlebell.

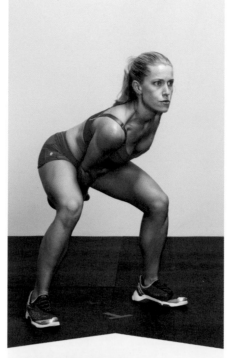

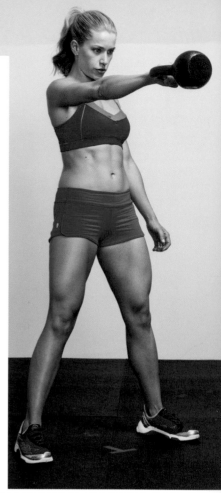

ONE-HANDED SWING
Follow the instructions for the two-handed swing, except hold the weight in one hand at a time.

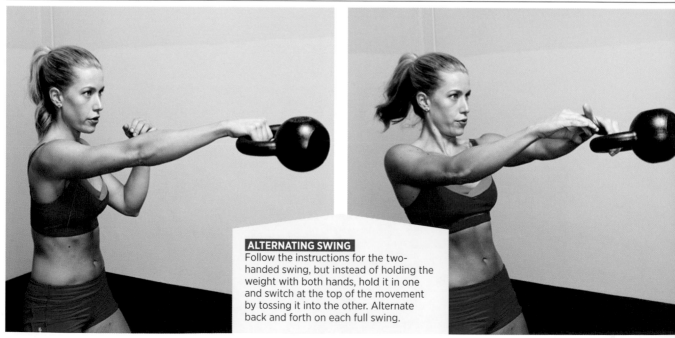

ALTERNATING SWING
Follow the instructions for the two-handed swing, but instead of holding the weight with both hands, hold it in one and switch at the top of the movement by tossing it into the other. Alternate back and forth on each full swing.

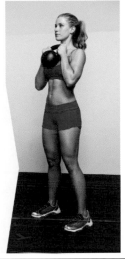

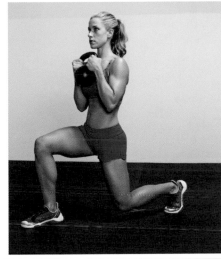

REVERSE LUNGE

GET READY: Holding a kettlebell at chest level, step backward with your left foot from a standing position into a lunge.

GO: Bend both knees to lower your hips toward the floor, keeping your torso upright. Stop before your rear knee touches the floor and then return to a standing position. Repeat, this time stepping backward with your right foot. Alternate for reps.

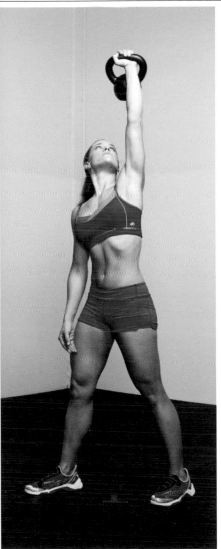

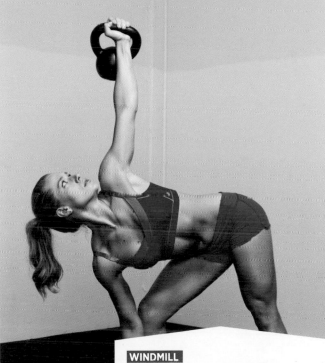

WINDMILL

GET READY: Stand with your feet shoulder-width apart and hold a kettlebell overhead with your left hand.

GO: With both eyes on the weight, lean sideways at the hips as you keep your arm in the overhead vertical position. Touch your right hand to your right foot, making sure that arm is perfectly straight. (At the bottom, your upper body will form a sideways lowercase T.) Slowly return to a standing position without dropping the weight and repeat the sequence one or two more times before switching arms.

KETTLE-BELLS TURN UP THE HEAT

Wondering how kettlebell training can benefit your pursuit of an athletic physique? Kirsten Farrell, an RKC-certified trainer in Venice, CA, points out that regularly working out with kettlebells improves muscular strength, bone density, and cardiovascular fitness.

Also, when done properly, kettlebell exercises hit all aspects of the core, she points out. "This is especially beneficial to women after pregnancy who are working to get their pre-baby body back."

In addition, kettlebell training activates many muscle groups at once to ramp up the body's fat-torching abilities. "All women want the most bang for their buck when it comes to burning calories," Farrell notes. "A good kettlebell workout will prompt the body to continue burning calories at a higher rate not only during exercise, but afterward, too."

Throw, Jump, Lunge

Sculpt a lean, muscular hardbody with this effective medicine-ball circuit

THROW AND CHASE

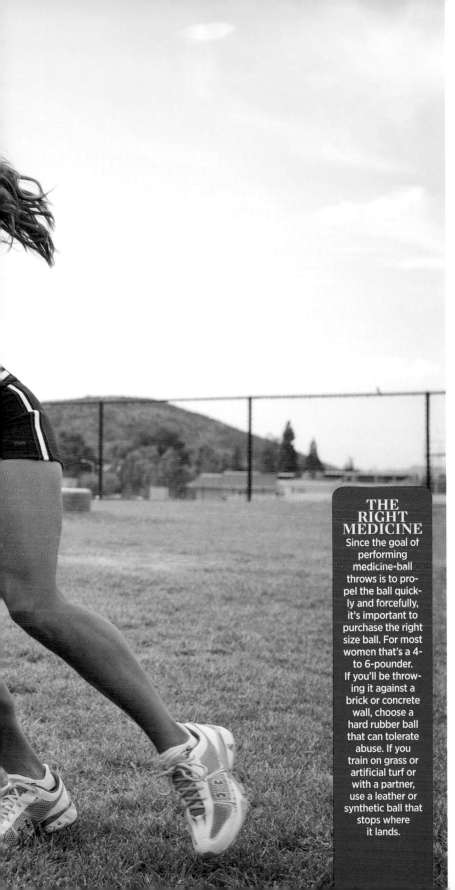

Chances are pretty good that you've held a medicine ball. You may have even used one while squatting, lunging, or twisting. But the chances are equally good that you've never realized the full potential of a med ball and you're skeptical of just how well these weighted spheres can produce real-world results.

If you've never trained in the great outdoors with one, then your skepticism is warranted. Because that's where these affordable, low-maintenance weights offer you the ability to perform a vast number of exercise combinations to burn fat, build strength, and inject much-needed variety into your routine.

"I use medicine-ball throws with all my clients," says Rachel Rose, former elite rower and New York personal trainer. "I've found that women love to get outside and do something less conventional than typical machine circuits, or treadmill or elliptical work."

The real advantage to taking these old-school tools outside is in the dynamic possibilities they offer. When you lift weights in the gym, the environment limits the speed and force with which you can move a free weight or machine handle. To generate maximum force on the bench press, for example, you'd need to throw the barbell or dumbbells into the air. But hurtling weights across the gym is fraught with all kinds of legal and physical implications.

Medicine balls taken outside, on the other hand, can be thrown with all the force you can muster, which means there's no limit to how much speed or effort you use. Simply put, you can train without constraint and from every conceivable angle. Athletes run, jump, and throw with freedom of movement, and that's the most effective way to train with medicine balls.

In fact, this focus on movement as opposed to isolated body parts can help give you that sleek, athletic look. This routine will teach you to move more fluidly, recruit more motor units, and use your entire body to complete a task, and it'll raise your heart rate using high-intensity interval training (HIIT), commonly regarded as the best way to burn fat.

"Athletes look great because they train athletically," Rose says. "This sounds obvious, but it's not because most people don't know how athletes train. Medicine balls are a staple for elite athletes, and they're so versatile that any woman can incorporate them into her program."

THE RIGHT MEDICINE

Since the goal of performing medicine-ball throws is to propel the ball quickly and forcefully, it's important to purchase the right size ball. For most women that's a 4- to 6-pounder. If you'll be throwing it against a brick or concrete wall, choose a hard rubber ball that can tolerate abuse. If you train on grass or artificial turf or with a partner, use a leather or synthetic ball that stops where it lands.

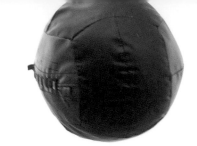

CHAPTER **8** Throw, Jump, Lunge

Medicine-Ball Circuit Training

This workout offers a comprehensive sampling of what's possible with medicine-ball training. You'll start with the throw and chase, a super full-body warmup that can be used for any sport. After that, you'll go through a series of HIIT-style movements designed to burn fat, build explosive power, and work various energy systems to get you in better overall shape. These moves are most effective when performed at the start of a session because your central nervous system is relatively untaxed and you can move the ball faster and more forcefully. Finally, you'll perform three strength-building exercises: the overhead walking lunge, medicine ball pushup, and push crunch.

EXERCISE	SETS	REPS	REST
Throw and Chase	2	100 yards	1 min.
Half-squat Jump Throw and Chase	1	10	1 min.
Half-squat Jump-Bounce Throw and Chase	1	10	1 min.
Backward Overhead Throw and Chase	1	10	1 min.
Side-twist Throw and Chase	1	10 each side	1 min.
Kneeling Coil Throw	1	10	1 min.
Overhead Walking Lunge	2	20 steps	1 min.
Medicine Ball Pushup	2	10 each side	1 min.
Medicine Ball Push Crunch	2	20	30 sec.

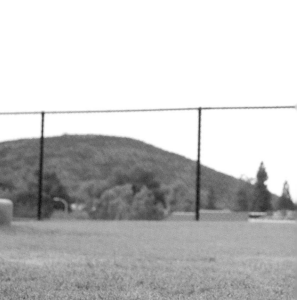

KNEELING COIL THROW

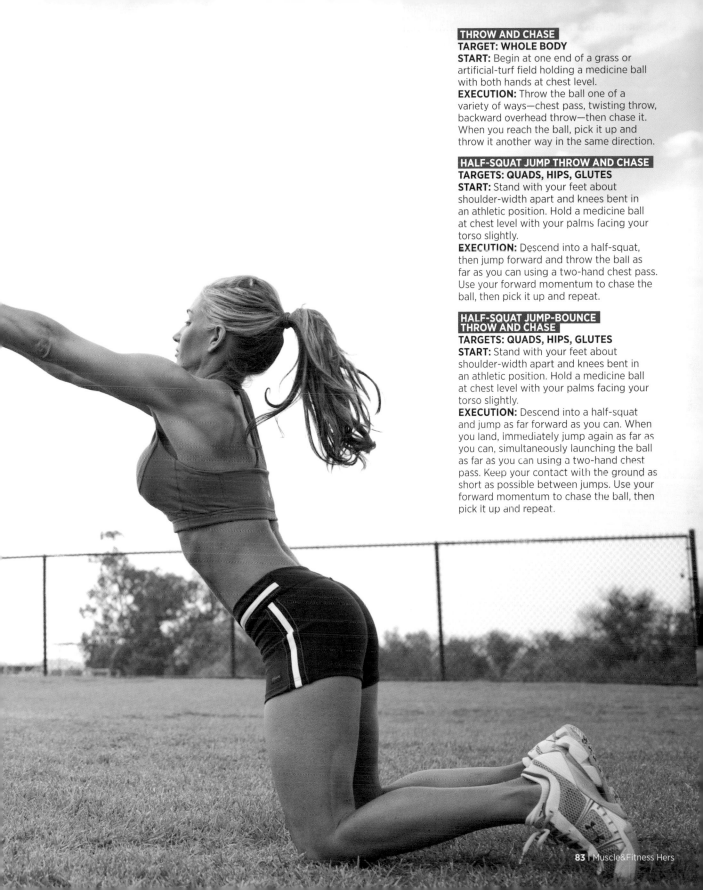

THROW AND CHASE
TARGET: WHOLE BODY
START: Begin at one end of a grass or artificial-turf field holding a medicine ball with both hands at chest level.
EXECUTION: Throw the ball one of a variety of ways—chest pass, twisting throw, backward overhead throw—then chase it. When you reach the ball, pick it up and throw it another way in the same direction.

HALF-SQUAT JUMP THROW AND CHASE
TARGETS: QUADS, HIPS, GLUTES
START: Stand with your feet about shoulder-width apart and knees bent in an athletic position. Hold a medicine ball at chest level with your palms facing your torso slightly.
EXECUTION: Descend into a half-squat, then jump forward and throw the ball as far as you can using a two-hand chest pass. Use your forward momentum to chase the ball, then pick it up and repeat.

HALF-SQUAT JUMP-BOUNCE THROW AND CHASE
TARGETS: QUADS, HIPS, GLUTES
START: Stand with your feet about shoulder-width apart and knees bent in an athletic position. Hold a medicine ball at chest level with your palms facing your torso slightly.
EXECUTION: Descend into a half-squat and jump as far forward as you can. When you land, immediately jump again as far as you can, simultaneously launching the ball as far as you can using a two-hand chest pass. Keep your contact with the ground as short as possible between jumps. Use your forward momentum to chase the ball, then pick it up and repeat.

BACKWARD OVERHEAD THROW AND CHASE

TARGETS: HAMSTRINGS, LOWER BACK

START: With your feet slightly wider than shoulder width, squat down and hold a medicine ball with both hands between your legs.

EXECUTION: Extend your knees, hips, and arms, and throw the ball as high and as far behind you as you can. Turn and chase it, pick it up and repeat.

SIDE-TWIST THROW AND CHASE

TARGETS: HIPS, OBLIQUES

START: Stand erect with your feet slightly wider than shoulder width and your toes pointed forward. Hold a medicine ball at chest level, arms extended.

EXECUTION: Twist as far to one side as you can, then toss the ball as far as you can to the opposite side as you rotate that direction. Chase the ball, then pick it up and repeat to the opposite side. Make sure you propel the ball using your torso, not your arms or hands.

KNEELING COIL THROW

TARGETS: QUADS, CHEST, TRICEPS

START: Kneel on the ground holding a medicine ball at chest level with your palms facing your torso slightly.

EXECUTION: Using a two-hand chest pass, throw the ball as far as you can and land in a pushup position. Retrieve the ball and repeat. If you perform this movement against a wall, push off the wall back to a kneeling position, retrieve the ball and repeat. If you work with a partner, have her roll the ball back to you.

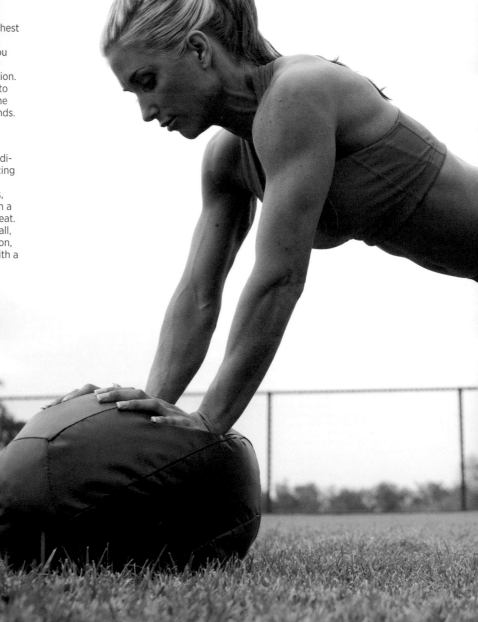

MEDICINE BALL PUSHUP

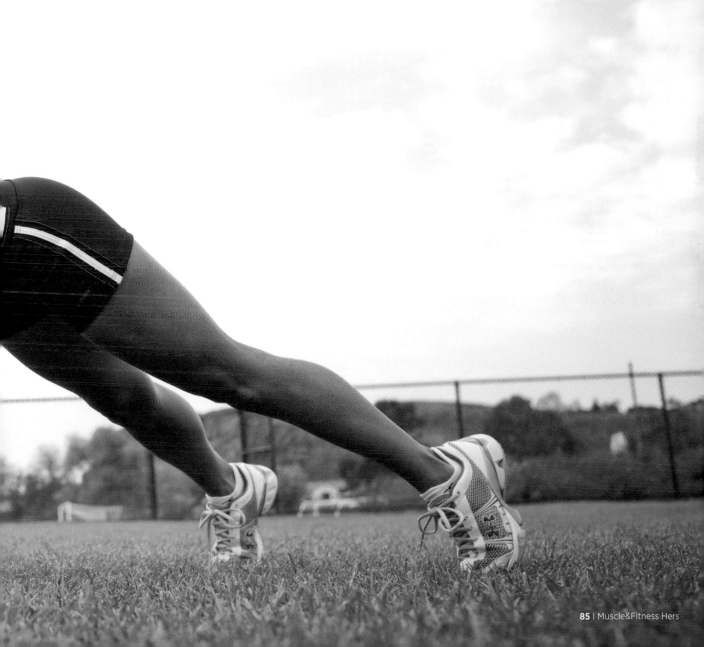

OVERHEAD WALKING LUNGE
TARGETS: QUADS, GLUTES

START: Stand erect with your feet shoulder-width apart holding a medicine ball in front of you with both hands.

EXECUTION: Raise the ball overhead and step forward into a lunge. Descend until your front knee forms a 90-degree angle and your back knee nearly touches the ground. Lower the ball to waist level and drive through your front foot to bring your back leg forward and return to standing. Repeat with the opposite leg in front.

MEDICINE BALL PUSHUP
TARGETS: CHEST, SHOULDERS, TRICEPS

START: Get in pushup position with your hands near a medicine ball.

EXECUTION: Place one hand on the ball and one on the ground, and perform a pushup. Reverse your hand position and repeat, alternating hands for reps.

MEDICINE BALL PUSH CRUNCH
TARGET: ABS

START: Lie faceup with your knees bent about 90 degrees and your feet flat on the ground. Hold a medicine ball with both hands, arms extended directly above your face.

EXECUTION: Keeping the ball above you, contract your abs to raise your upper body off the ground. Hold for a second, then return to the start position.

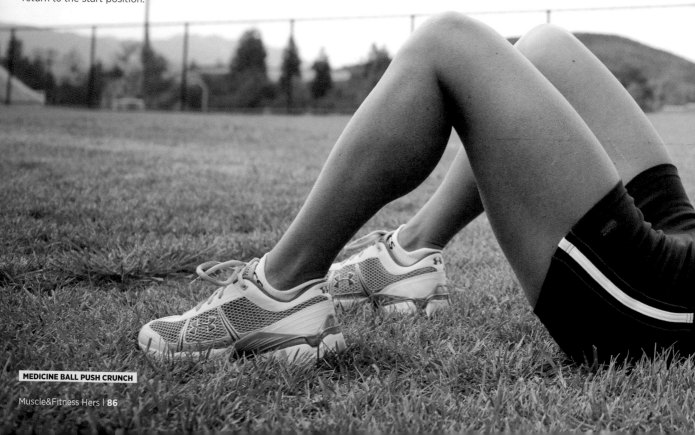

MEDICINE BALL PUSH CRUNCH

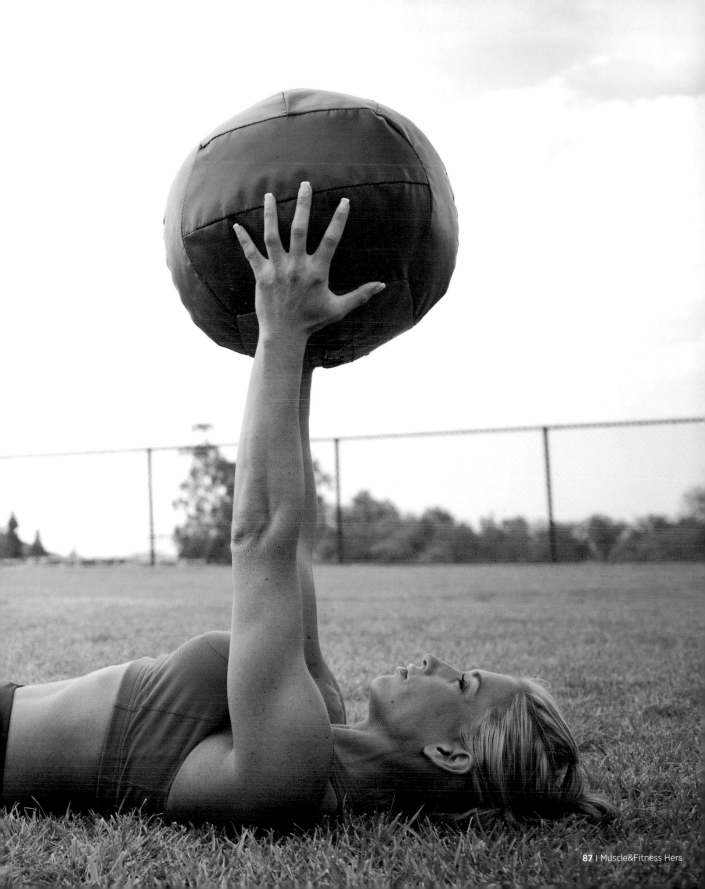

CHAPTER 9

Home for the Holidays

Is the gift of stress-free fitness this holiday season music to your ears? These *Hers* home workouts are designed to keep your training goals on target, no matter how chaotic your calendar gets.

It's never too early to start planning for the holiday season—and for all the commitments that come with it. Like family get-togethers, awkward work functions, decorating, cooking, wrapping, and shuttling the kids between visits with the mall Santa and their not-quite-ready-for-primetime school plays. Did we mention shopping?

Yes, November and December can mean a total derailment of your fitness efforts. Health clubs across the country empty faster than a Saks sales rack as people trade dumbbells for hors d'oeuvres and treadmills for teeming Target parking lots.

As a fitness enthusiast, you have two choices around the holidays. You can harbor visions of juggling your regular workout schedule and those competing commitments with all the choreography of the New York City Ballet's Nutcracker production, most likely failing miserably in the process. Or you can use the *Hers* stress-free approach, bringing your workouts home for the holidays with one—or all three of our high-powered full-body training plans.

Each workout makes use of compound movements—exercises that incorporate multiple muscle groups, for maximum efficiency—and is designed for speed, so you can finish in 30 minutes without compromising your results.

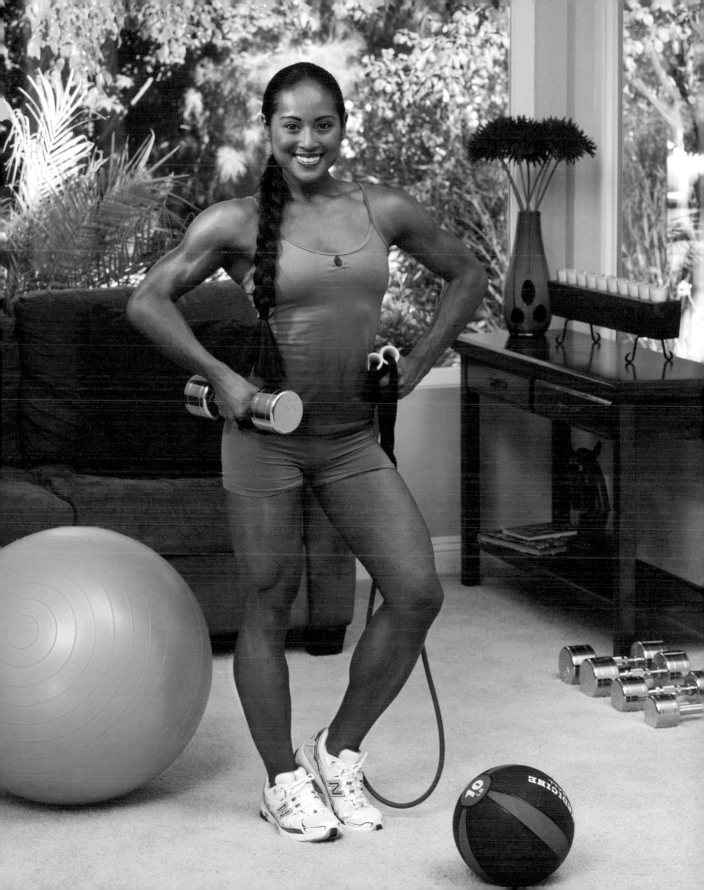

LEVEL 1: O COUNT ALL YE FAITHFUL

Our first barebones workout incorporates little equipment—all you'll need is a medicine ball and an open space—and makes use of high-intensity interval training (HIIT). Instead of counting reps, you simply do as many reps as you can in 20 seconds, then rest 10 seconds before moving on to the next exercise. Repeat the circuit four to eight times.

As you get more proficient at this workout, you can bump up your interval to a 30 seconds on 15 seconds' rest, and after that a 40/20 interval. According to Jim Stoppani, Ph.D., the most effective HIIT intervals for fat loss are ones that use a 2:1 work-to-rest ratio, which this program does.

EQUIPMENT CHECKLIST:
10–15-pound medicine ball ($12–$80)

THE WORKOUT
1/ Jump Squat
2/ Medicine Ball Single-leg Deadlift with Row Combo (20 seconds each side)
3/ Mountain Climber
4/ Walking Lunge with Ball Torso Twist
5/ Alternating Lunge Jump
6/ Medicine Ball Squat/Press/Curl Combo
7/ Jumping Jack
8/ Ball-roll Pushup
9/ Overhead Ball Crunch
10/ Burpee

JUMP SQUAT

> Stand in a shoulder-width stance, knees slightly bent, with both hands directly in front of you.
> Squat until your thighs approach parallel to the floor, then explode upward to leap in the air.
> Land with knees bent and return to the squat position immediately to reload for the next jump.

MEDICINE BALL SINGLE-LEG DEADLIFT WITH ROW COMBO

> Standing upright, hold a medicine ball in both hands. Both feet are on the floor in a stance just inside shoulder width.
> Hinging at your hips and keeping your upper back aligned with your core, bend over while balancing on one leg, lowering the ball to the floor with arms outstretched as the other leg rises behind you.
> When your upper body reaches nearly parallel to the floor, row the ball to your chest by bending both elbows, then lower it to full elbow extension and stand up.

MOUNTAIN CLIMBER

> Start in a modified pushup position, with your rear end elevated.
> Bring one knee in toward your chest.
> From here, energetically push up off your feet so they leave the floor and switch positions so the back foot comes forward and the front foot goes back.
> Continue jumping and alternating your foot position as quickly as you can, making sure your hands remain in contact with the floor throughout

WALKING LUNGE WITH BALL TORSO TWIST

> Stand holding a medicine ball with both hands in front of your stomach.
> Step forward with one foot and bend both knees to lower your hips toward the floor as you twist your upper body toward the front-leg side.
> Return to a standing position, then step forward with the other foot while twisting to the opposite direction.
> Continue down the floor, alternating your lead leg and which way you twist.

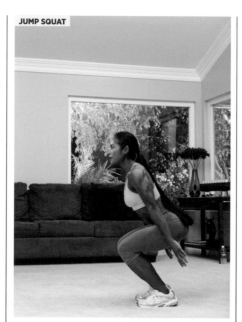

JUMP SQUAT

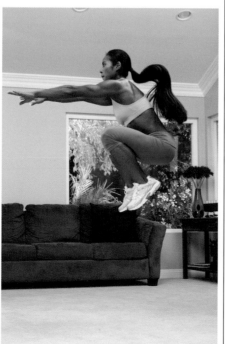

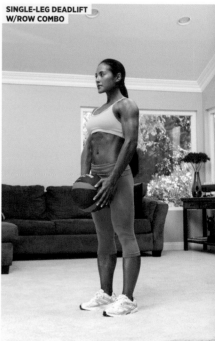

SINGLE-LEG DEADLIFT W/ROW COMBO

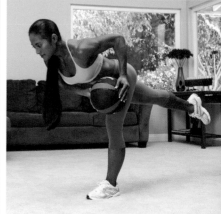

MOUNTAIN CLIMBER

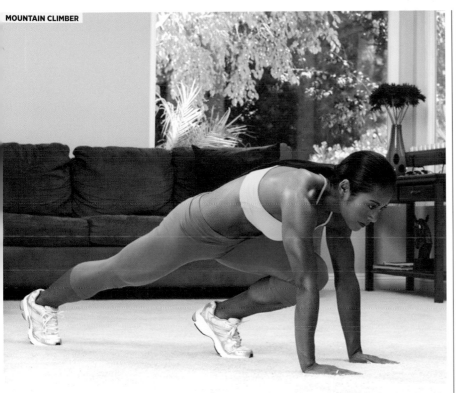

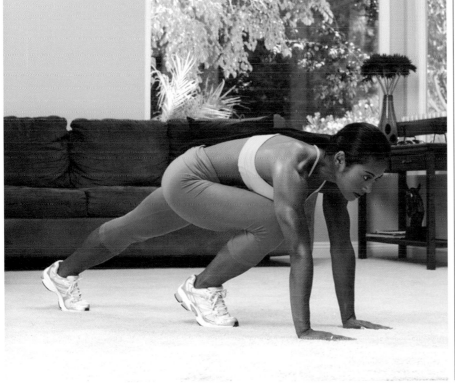

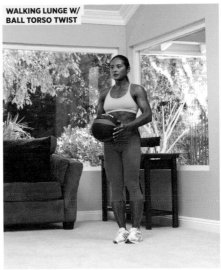

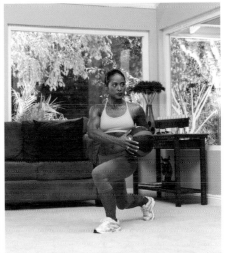

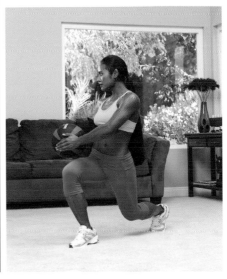

BURPEE

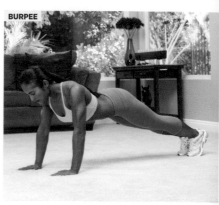

ALTERNATING LUNGE JUMP

> Step into a lunge position, one leg forward, one back, both knees bent, and torso upright.
> Dip down until your lead leg is at 90 degrees, then drive yourself upward off of the floor, switching leg position midair.
> Land with soft knees with the opposite legs forward and back.
> Repeat rapidly, reversing into the leap as soon as you reach the full lunge position.

MEDICINE BALL SQUAT/PRESS/CURL COMBO

> Hold a medicine ball in front of your chest.
> Squat down and lower the ball down between your legs. When the ball comes within a few inches of the floor, reverse the motion and stand, lifting the ball overhead.
> Go right into the next squat, and when you come up, keep your elbows at your sides and perform a curling motion with your arms.
> Alternate between the overhead press and the curl on each squatting repetition.

JUMPING JACK (NOT SHOWN)

BALL-ROLL PUSHUP

> Assume the pushup position on the floor, with one hand on a medicine ball.
> Keeping your head neutral and core tight, lower yourself toward the floor by bending your elbows, then extend your elbows fully to return to the start.
> At the top, roll the ball across to your other hand, and repeat.
> Roll the ball back and forth with each rep.

OVERHEAD BALL CRUNCH

> Lie faceup with your legs bent and your feet flat on the floor.
> Hold a medicine ball overhead with both hands, elbows alongside your ears—it will stay overhead throughout.
> Slowly curl your upper body off the floor, flex your abs for a moment, then lower and repeat, making sure not to lie back all the way down between reps.

BURPEE

> From a standing position, drop into a deep squat and contact the floor with your hands.
> Kick your feet back behind you, assume a plank position, perform a pushup, and quickly pull your feet back into the squat.
> Drive through your heels, leap up, land on soft knees and immediately descend into the squat to do the next rep.

ALTERNATING LUNGE JUMP

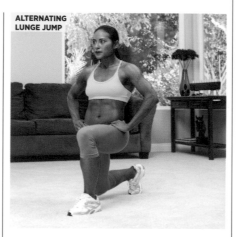

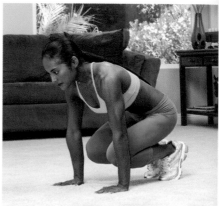

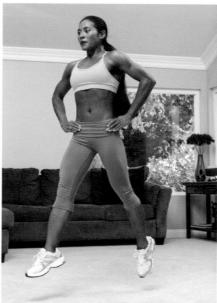

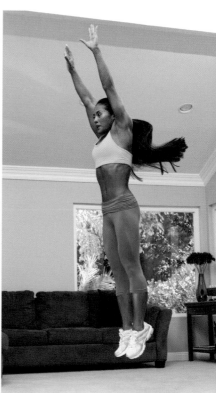

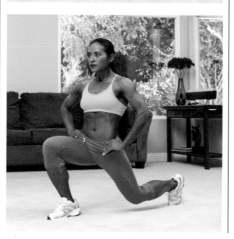

BALL-ROLL PUSHUP

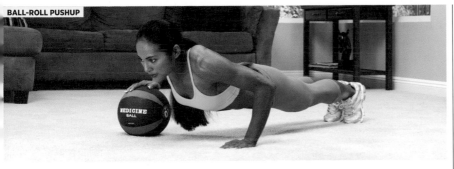

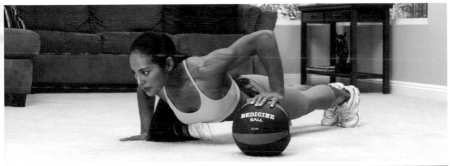

OVERHEAD BALL CRUNCH

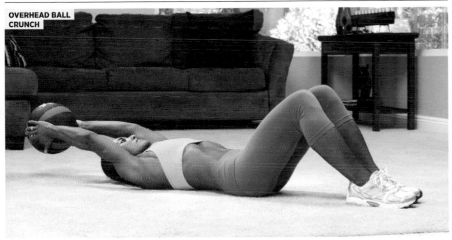

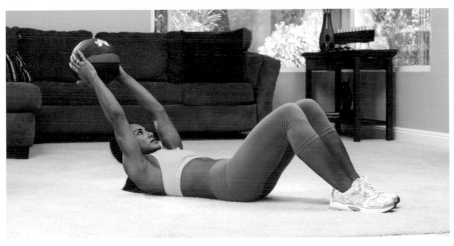

SQUAT/PRESS/CURL COMBO

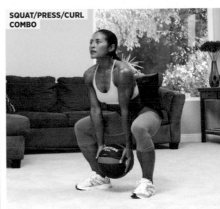

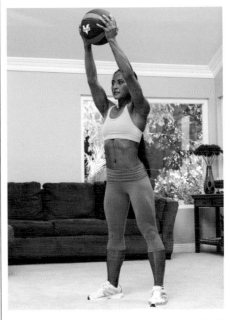

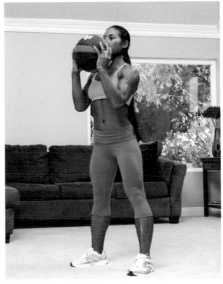

LEVEL 2: WINTER WONDER-BAND

A step up from our first option, this superset workout makes use of two conveniently packed pieces of equipment—bands and a jump rope—making it the perfect option for those times when you're on the road—provided the in-laws leave you alone for 20 minutes or so. Complete the paired exercises back to back with no rest in between, doing 10–15 reps per set. After you complete the superset, jump rope for 30–60 seconds, resting only if necessary between supersets. Repeat each superset three to five times before moving on to the next.

SQUAT

> Stand on the band with your feet approximately shoulder-width apart, holding the handles at the end of the bands in each hand.
> Shift your hips back and lower yourself into a squat position until your thighs are parallel to the floor.
> Push through your heels to until your knees are fully extended.

ALTERNATING OVERHEAD PRESS

> Stand with your hands at shoulder level holding the handles of the bands, elbows pointed down.
> Raise one arm overhead to full elbow extension, then lower and raise the other arm overhead; that's one rep.
> Keep the rest of your body still and your core tight, being sure not to lean back and forth as you raise the handle of the band overhead.

ROMANIAN DEADLIFT

> Stand upright with the band under your feet and a handle in each hand.
> Wrap the bands around your hands and hold the handle to increase tension.
> Keeping your core tight and back flat, lean forward, pushing your hips back until your torso is roughly parallel to the floor and your hands are near your feet.
> Pull your hips forward and squeeze your hamstrings, keeping your back flat as you return up.

LUNGE WITH LEG LIFT

> Place your front foot on the band.
> Keeping your upper body erect, sink down on your front leg until it is parallel to the floor. Push up through your heel to stand up.
> As you do, keep your back leg in a locked position, knee slightly bent, and lift it up off the floor, squeezing your ham and glute for a two-count.
> Repeat, then switch legs.

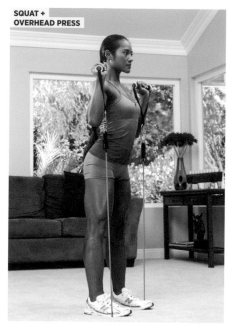

SQUAT +
OVERHEAD PRESS

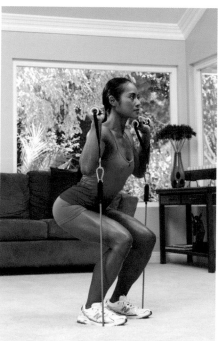

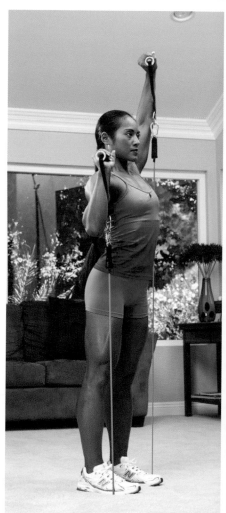

EQUIPMENT CHECKLIST:
*Resistance bands ($45–$130)**
Jump rope ($5–$25)
*Bands sold at bodylastics.com

THE WORKOUT

1/ *Superset #1*
Squat + Alternating Overhead Press
2/ *Superset #2*
Romanian Deadlift + Lunge with Leg Lift
3/ *Superset #3*
Straight-arm Pulldown + Band Flye
4/ *Superset #4*
Overhead Triceps Extension + Biceps Curl
5/ *Superset #5*
Reverse Crunch + Crunch*

Jump rope for 30 seconds after completing each superset.
**Perform each for one minute, with no rest in between.*

ROMANIAN DEADLIFT

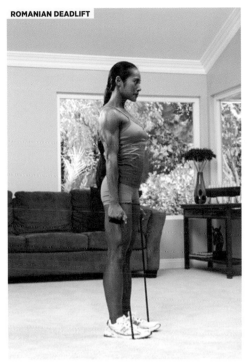

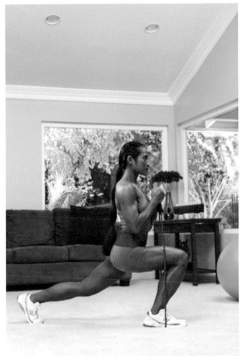

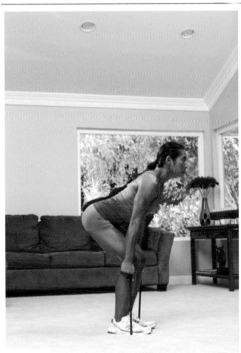

LUNGE W/LEG LIFT

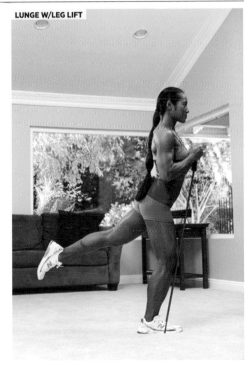

STRAIGHT-ARM PULLDOWN

> Anchor the midpoint of the band at the top of a door, face the door with a handle in each hand, palms facing behind you.
> Remove slack from the band with both arms above your head.
> Elbows straight, bring your arms as far behind you as you can.
> Squeeze for a two-count, then return to the starting position.

+

BAND FLYE

> Face away from the door and step forward to remove slack from the band, holding a handle in each hand.
> Extend your arms out to your sides and bend your elbows, so the handles are roughly even with your chest.
> Push the bands forward in a wide arc.
> When your hands meet, squeeze your chest for a two-count.
> Slowly return to the starting position along the same arc.

OVERHEAD TRICEPS EXTENSION

> Stand with your feet atop the band, grasping a handle in each hand, and bring your arms up so your elbows are alongside your ears.
> Moving only at your elbows, extend your arms straight above you.
> Squeeze your triceps tight, then lower and repeat.

+

BICEPS CURL

> Stand with your arms at your sides holding the handles, feet atop the cable.
> Moving only at your elbows and keeping them in place at your sides, curl the handles toward your upper body.
> Squeeze your biceps, and then lower to full extension and repeat.

REVERSE CRUNCH

+

CRUNCH

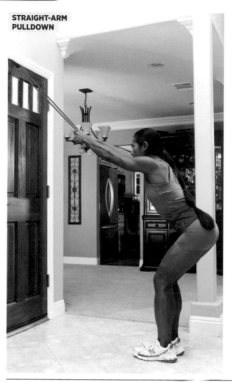
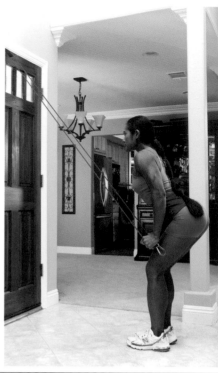

STRAIGHT-ARM PULLDOWN

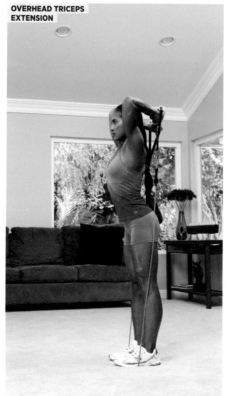
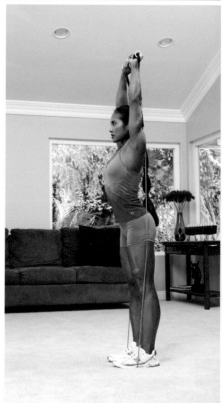

OVERHEAD TRICEPS EXTENSION

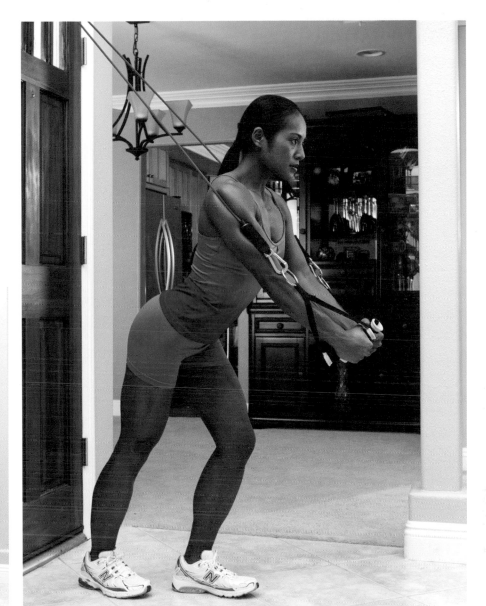

BAND FLYE

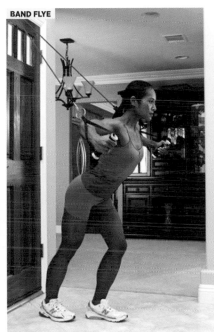

REVERSE CRUNCH + CRUNCH

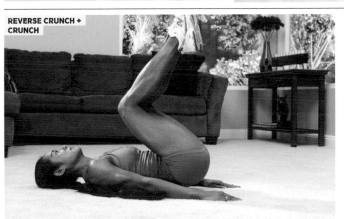

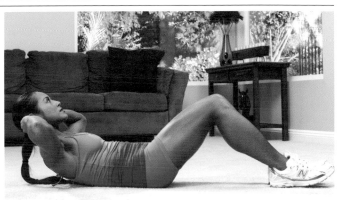

LEVEL 3: HOLIDAY HIIT LIST

Our platinum option is more costly than the previous two, but your body will thank you for it if you have the means. This plan divides the body into two resistance-based workouts broken up with short durations of HIIT cardio sessions in order to get your heart rate up and your body into fat-burning mode during your workout. You'll also add one cardio-only session on of one the nonworkout days. For each exercise listed, you'll perform three sets of 8–12 repetitions, using the heaviest dumbbell you can handle with good form on each.

TREADMILL

BALL WALL SQUAT (NOT SHOWN)

> Stand against an exercise ball that's placed between you and a wall; the ball should be at your lower back to start.
> Lower yourself straight down as if you're about to sit in a chair by lowering your hips and bending both knees, rolling the ball along the wall.
> When your thighs reach a point parallel to the floor or slightly below, push through your heels to stand up.

REVERSE DUMBBELL LUNGE

> Stand holding a dumbbell in each hand.
> Keeping your upper body upright, step backward with one leg, and sink your hips to the floor, bringing your back knee close to the ground.
> Stop just short of your rear knee touching the floor, then drive yourself forward, bringing your rear foot forward into another lunge position.
> Repeat for reps, then switch legs.

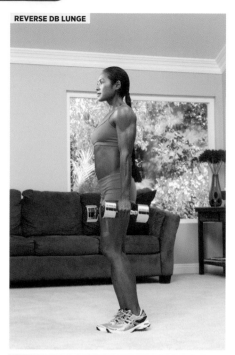

REVERSE DB LUNGE

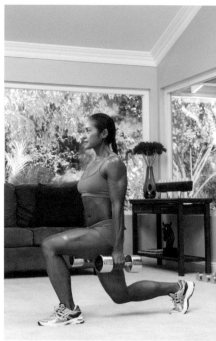

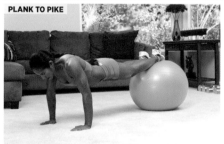

PLANK TO PIKE

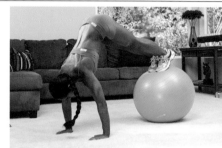

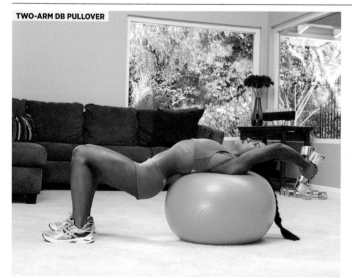

TWO-ARM DB PULLOVER

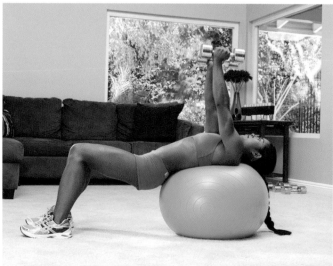

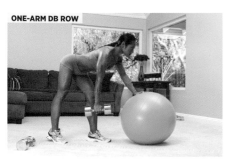
ONE-ARM DB ROW

WORKOUT 1: BACK/LEGS/CORE
1/ Treadmill (5-minute walk/light jog)
2/ Ball Wall Squat
3/ Reverse Dumbbell Lunge
4/ Ball Jump Squat
5/ Treadmill Sprints on Incline
(5 sprints, 30 seconds)
6/ One-arm Dumbbell Row on Ball
7/ Two-arm Dumbbell Pullover on Ball
8/ Treadmill Sprints on Flat Setting
(5 sprints, 30 seconds)
9/ Plank to Pike on Ball
10/ Back Extension on Ball

EQUIPMENT CHECKLIST:
Dumbbell set – 12, 15, 20 lbs ($25–$100)
Stability ball ($20–$45))
Treadmill ($120–$2,000)

Weekly Training Split

MONDAY	WORKOUT 1
TUESDAY	WORKOUT 2
WEDNESDAY	OFF
THURSDAY	WORKOUT 1
FRIDAY	WORKOUT 2
SATURDAY	CARDIO (45 TO 90 MINUTES)

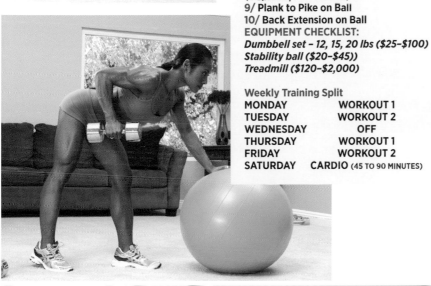

BALL JUMP SQUAT (NOT SHOWN)
> Holding an exercise ball in front of your body with both hands, lower your hips to the floor by bending your knees into a squat position.
> Touch the ball down to the floor in front of you, then drive through your heels to jump into the air, extending the ball above you.
> Land on "soft" knees (slightly bent), return to a squat position and jump again.

ONE-ARM DUMBBELL ROW ON BALL
> Bend at the waist and place one hand on a ball, holding a dumbbell with a neutral grip and arm extended.
> With your back flat and core tight, pull the weight toward your hip and squeeze for a two-count, keeping your elbow close to your side throughout the movement.
> Lower the dumbbell along the same path. Repeat for reps, then switch arms.

TWO-ARM DUMBBELL PULLOVER ON BALL
> Lie faceup on a ball, holding a dumbbell in each hand with your arms extended above your chest.
> Keeping a slight bend in your elbows, lower the dumbbells behind your head.
> When you feel the pull in your lats, lift the dumbbells back along the same path to the starting position.

PLANK TO PIKE ON BALL
> Get into a pushup position with your shins on the exercise ball and hands on the floor.
> From that plank position, raise into a pike by lifting your butt toward the ceiling, which in turn will roll the ball from your shins to your toes.
> Lower yourself back to a plank and repeat for reps.

BACK EXTENSION ON BALL
> Place the ball under your hips with your knees straight, legs together, toes on the floor, and hands behind your head.
> Anchor yourself by putting your heels against a wall.
> From a position where your body is straight from your feet to your head, lower your torso toward the ball by bending at the hips.
> Lift your chest off the ball to return to the fully aligned position.

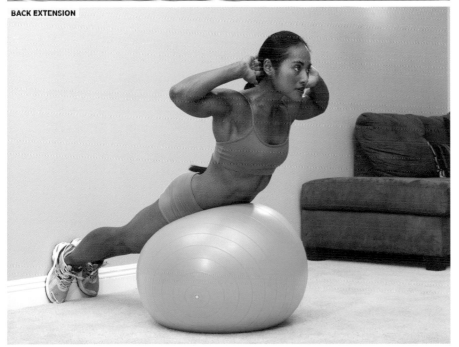
BACK EXTENSION

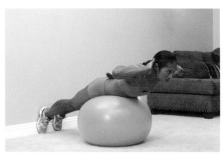

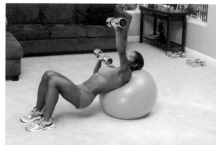

INCLINE ALTERNATING DB PRESS

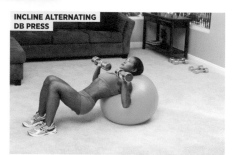

WORKOUT 2: CHEST/SHOULDERS/ARMS

1/ Treadmill (5 minute walk/light jog)
2/ Incline Alternating Dumbbell Press on Ball
3/ Flat Dumbbell Flye on Ball
4/ Pushup on Ball
5/ Treadmill Sprints on Incline (5 sprints, 30 seconds)
6/ Seated Dumbbell Press on Ball
7/ Dumbbell Lateral Raise
8/ Treadmill Sprints on Flat Setting (5 sprints, 30 seconds)
9/ Seated Alternating Curl on Ball
10/ Lying Triceps Extension on Ball
11/ Treadmill Sprints on Flat Setting (5 sprints, 20 seconds)

TREADMILL

INCLINE ALTERNATING DUMBBELL PRESS ON BALL

> Lie on the ball so that your upper back is supported; your knees bent so you're at an incline position (as if you were on an incline bench).
> Hold a pair of dumbbells at chest level.
> Press one dumbbell upward toward the ceiling, keeping the other at chest level.
> Slowly lower one dumbbell and, as you reach chest level, press the other toward the ceiling.
> Repeat for reps.

FLAT DUMBBELL FLYE ON BALL

> Lie faceup on the ball with your feet flat on the floor, holding a dumbbell just outside your shoulder in each hand with a neutral grip.
> Extend your arms above your chest, then slowly lower the dumbbells in a wide arc out to your sides, keeping your elbows locked in a slightly bent position throughout the range of motion.
> Stop when your elbows reach shoulder level and reverse the motion.

PUSHUP ON BALL (NOT SHOWN)

> Lie facedown with your thighs on the ball, feet straight out and in line with your head and spine, and your hands on the floor in a pushup position.
> Lower your body by bending your elbows as far as you can, then extend your elbows to return to the start.

SEATED DUMBBELL PRESS ON BALL

> Sit on the ball, holding a dumbbell in each hand at shoulder level with palms facing forward.
> Keep your head straight, eyes focused forward and your shoulders back, and press the dumbbells overhead in an arc, stopping just before the weights touch at the top.
> Slowly lower the dumbbells to shoulder level and repeat.

DUMBBELL LATERAL RAISE

> Stand with your feet shoulder-width apart, your abs tight, chest up, and shoulders back;

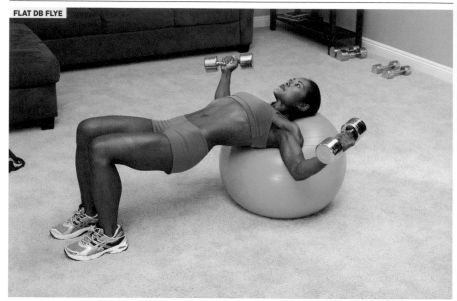

FLAT DB FLYE

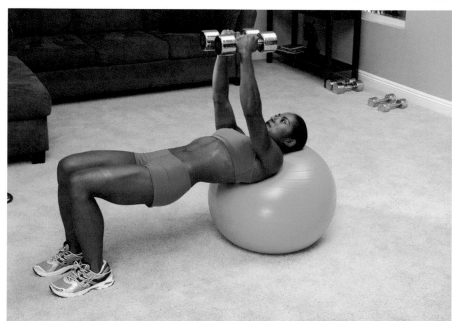

SEATED DB PRESS

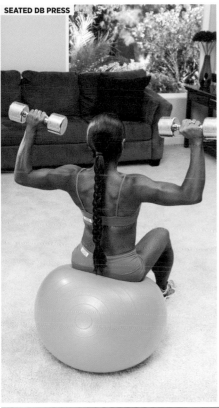

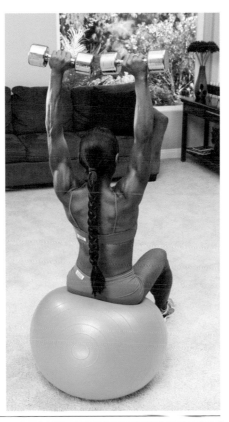

and hold dumbbells at your sides with a neutral grip.
> Raise the dumbbells out to your sides in a wide arc, keeping your elbows and hands moving together in the same plane, until they reach shoulder level.
> Hold the weights momentarily in the peak-contracted position and slowly lower them along the same path, stopping before they come in contact with your sides before beginning the next rep.

SEATED ALTERNATING CURL ON BALL

> Sit on the ball, holding a dumbbell in each hand at your sides.
> Keeping your chest up, curl one dumbbell up toward the same-side shoulder, squeezing your biceps hard at the top, then lower to the start.
> Repeat with the other arm.

LYING TRICEPS EXTENSION ON BALL

> Lie faceup on the ball, holding a dumbbell in each hand, raise them above your chest, arms angled slightly backward.
> Bending just at the elbows, and keeping your upper arms in a locked position, lower the dumbbells behind your head, to about forehead level.
> Slowly return the dumbbells to the starting position, squeezing your triceps at the top of the movement.

LYING TRICEPS EXTENSION

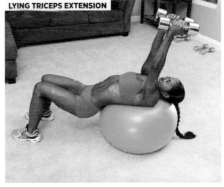

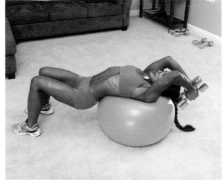

DB LATERAL RAISE

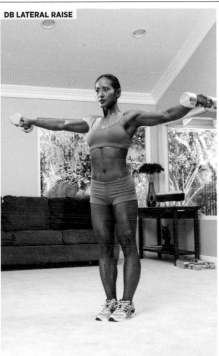

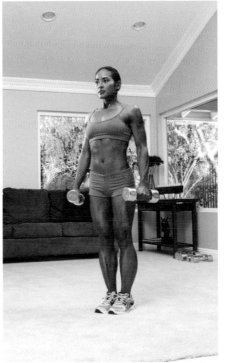

The Vacation Workout

Stay in shape when you're on the road with three fast, effective workouts

N ow that you've seen our crash course from Chapter 9 on how to stay in shape over the holidays, what about staying in shape while you're away from home on vacation? We've got you covered with three quick and effective total-body workouts that combine resistance and cardiovascular training. All you need is a set of resistance bands and voilà: Your gym comes to you, wherever you are.

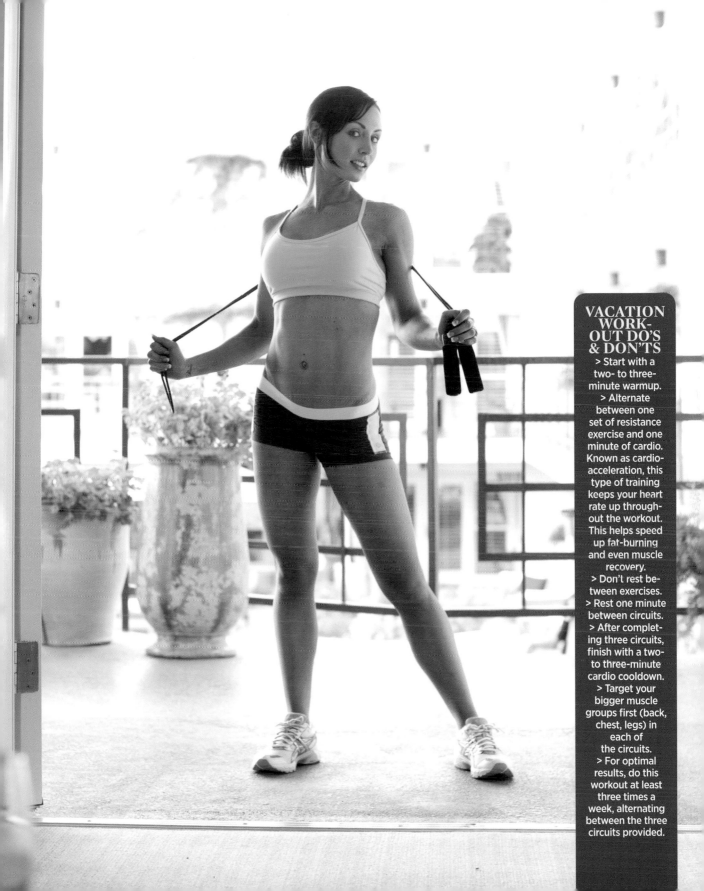

Circuit 1

MUSCLE GROUP	EXERCISE	REPS/TIME
(Warmup)	Jog in Place	2–3 min.
Chest	Decline Pushup	To failure
	Jog in Place	1 min.
Legs	Squat	10–12
	Jog in Place	1 min.
Back	One-arm Bentover Row	12–15
	Jog in Place	1 min.
Shoulders	Overhead Press	12–15
	Jog in Place	1 min.
Biceps	Standing Curl	12–15
	Jog in Place	1 min.
Triceps	Overhead Triceps Extension	12–15
	Jog in Place	1 min.
Abs	Crunch	To failure
	Jog in Place	1 min.

Don't rest between exercises. Rest one minute between circuits. After three circuits, finish with a two- to three-minute cooldown.

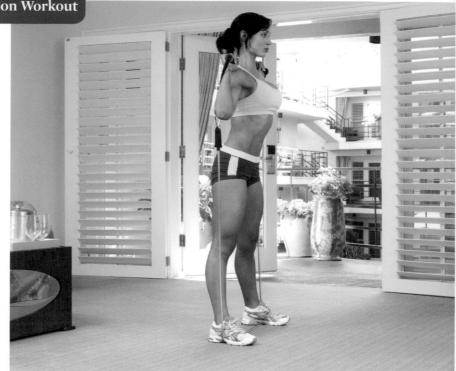

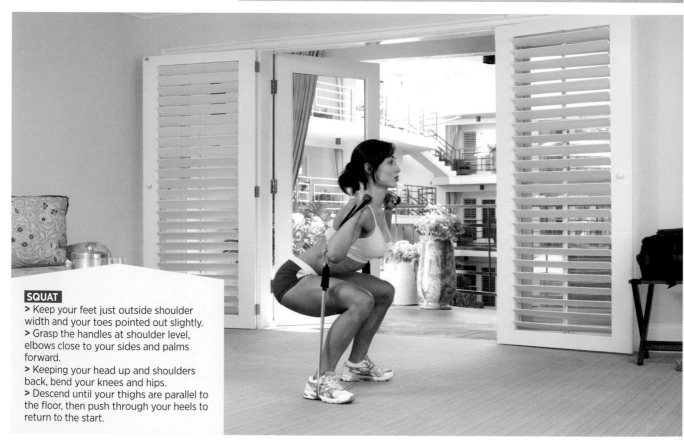

SQUAT
> Keep your feet just outside shoulder width and your toes pointed out slightly.
> Grasp the handles at shoulder level, elbows close to your sides and palms forward.
> Keeping your head up and shoulders back, bend your knees and hips.
> Descend until your thighs are parallel to the floor, then push through your heels to return to the start.

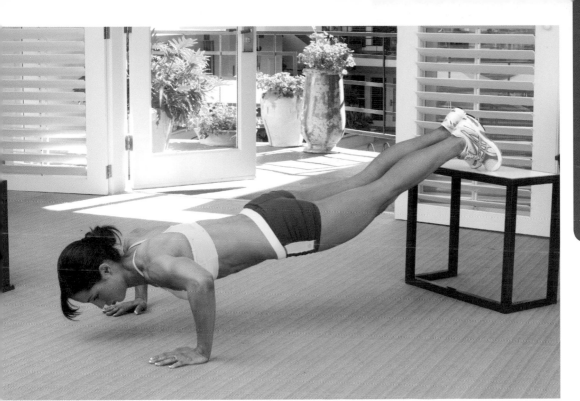

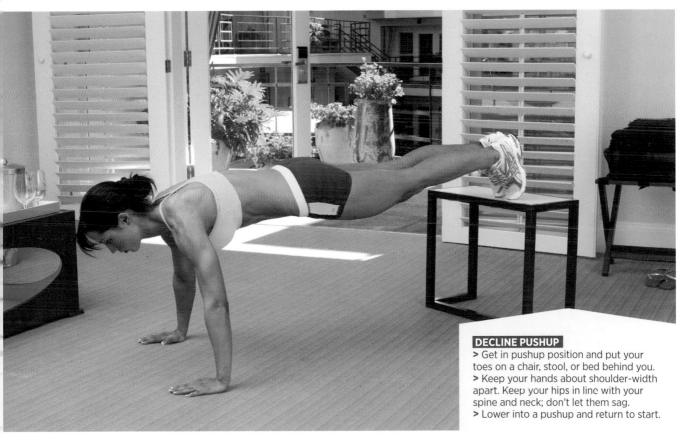

DECLINE PUSHUP

> Get in pushup position and put your toes on a chair, stool, or bed behind you.
> Keep your hands about shoulder-width apart. Keep your hips in line with your spine and neck; don't let them sag.
> Lower into a pushup and return to start.

Circuit 2

MUSCLE GROUP	EXERCISE	REPS/TIME
(Warmup)	Jog in Place	2–3 min.
Chest	Pushup	To failure
	Jump Rope*	1 min.
Legs	Jump Squat	To failure
	Jump Rope*	1 min.
Back	Lat Pulldown	10–12
	Jump Rope*	1 min.
Shoulders	Lateral Raise	10–12
	Jump Rope*	1 min.
Biceps	Behind-the-back Curl	10–12
	Jump Rope*	1 min.
Triceps	Chair Dip	To failure
	Jump Rope*	1 min.
Abs	Reverse Crunch	To failure
	Jump Rope*	1 min.

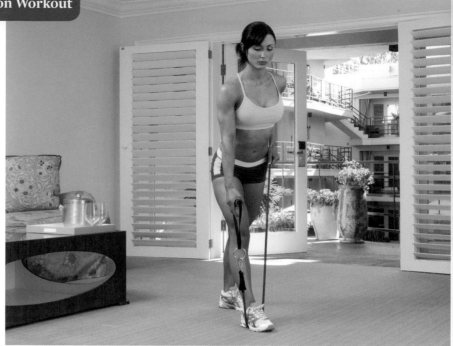

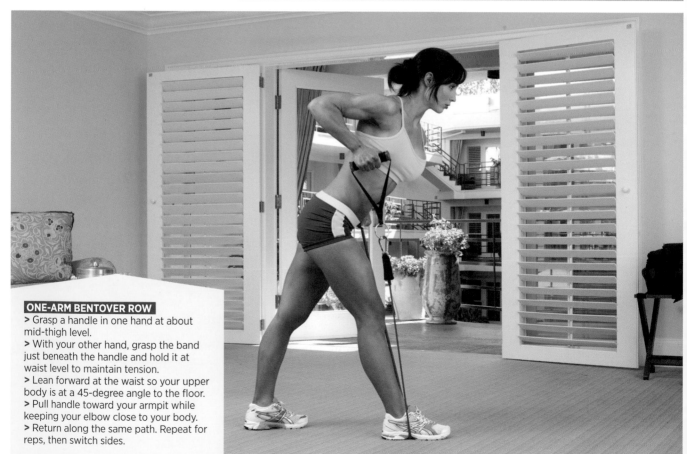

ONE-ARM BENTOVER ROW
> Grasp a handle in one hand at about mid-thigh level.
> With your other hand, grasp the band just beneath the handle and hold it at waist level to maintain tension.
> Lean forward at the waist so your upper body is at a 45-degree angle to the floor.
> Pull handle toward your armpit while keeping your elbow close to your body.
> Return along the same path. Repeat for reps, then switch sides.

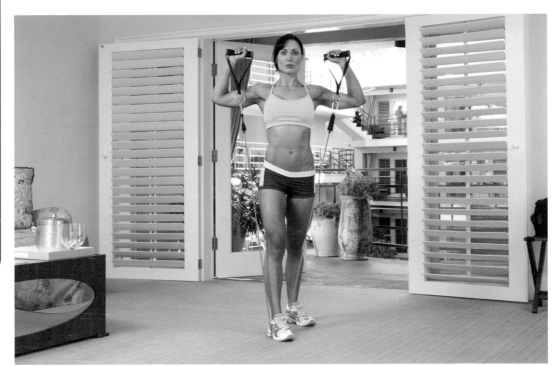

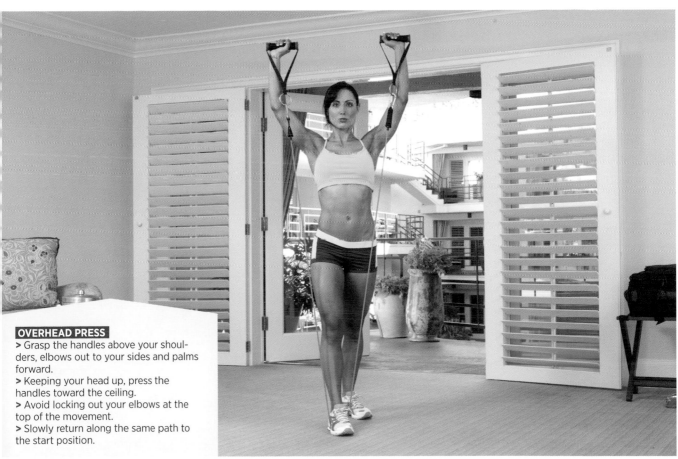

OVERHEAD PRESS

> Grasp the handles above your shoulders, elbows out to your sides and palms forward.
> Keeping your head up, press the handles toward the ceiling.
> Avoid locking out your elbows at the top of the movement.
> Slowly return along the same path to the start position.

Circuit 3

MUSCLE GROUP	EXERCISE	REPS/TIME
(Warmup)	Jog in Place	2–3 min.
Chest	Incline Pushup	To failure
	Burpee*	1 min.
Legs	Reverse Lunge	To failure
	Burpee*	1 min.
Back	Straight-arm Pulldown	8–10
	Burpee*	1 min.
Shoulders	Upright Row	8–10
	Burpee*	1 min.
Biceps	Reverse-grip Curl	8–10
	Burpee*	1 min.
Triceps	Close-grip Pushup	To failure
	Burpee*	1 min.
Abs	Plank	1 min.
	Burpee*	1 min.

Don't rest between exercises. Rest one minute between circuits. After completing three circuits, finish with a 2–3-minute cool-down.
*You can also do jumping jacks or run in place.

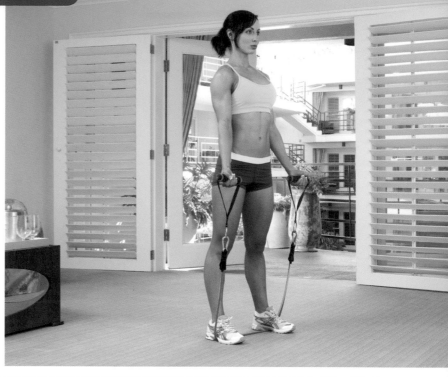

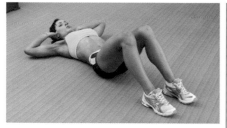

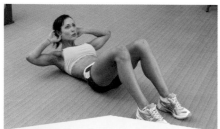

CRUNCH
> Lie faceup on the floor with your knees bent 90 degrees and your feet flat on the floor.
> Place your hands lightly behind your head or across your chest.
> Keep your chin up and your neck in line with your body; don't pull your head forward.
> Lift your shoulder blades off the floor and crunch toward your knees.

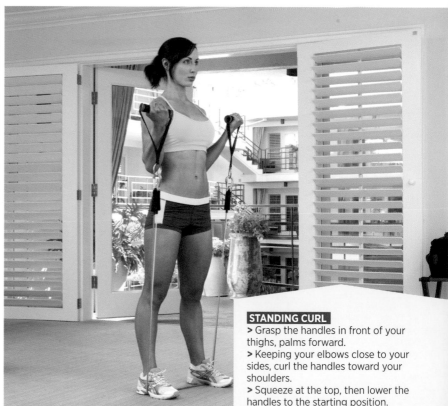

STANDING CURL
> Grasp the handles in front of your thighs, palms forward.
> Keeping your elbows close to your sides, curl the handles toward your shoulders.
> Squeeze at the top, then lower the handles to the starting position.

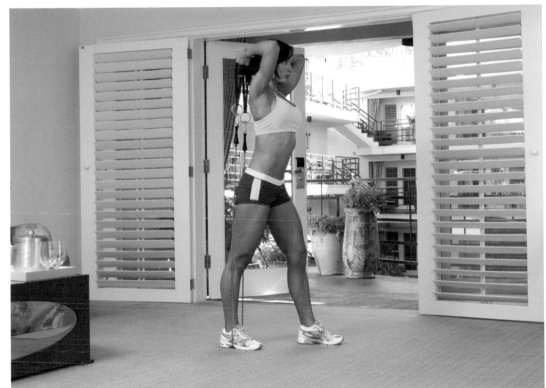

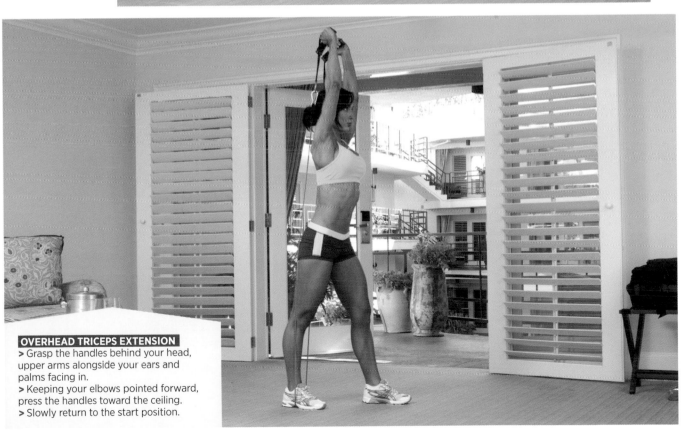

OVERHEAD TRICEPS EXTENSION

> Grasp the handles behind your head, upper arms alongside your ears and palms facing in.
> Keeping your elbows pointed forward, press the handles toward the ceiling.
> Slowly return to the start position.

Strike a Pose

Looking for a way to spice up your training while building muscle and burning fat? Try yoga.

It's a continual cycle: weight training to build muscle. Cardio to burn fat. For many *Hers* readers, that sequence takes place once or even twice a day, three, four, or five times a week. But if you're leaving regular yoga practice out of the loop, you could be shortchanging yourself in all kinds of ways.

Just ask Ariel Kiley, a yoga instructor in Los Angeles. Before discovering yoga, Kiley, a former actress (she had a short stint on *The Sopranos*) spent her time building muscle and trying to carve detail with the weights-and-cardio cycle, too—but without ever really getting the results she wanted.

"I knew I was physically fit. But for the amount of exercise I was doing, I was still pretty soft on top of the muscle I had built," she says. "When I started practicing yoga, the muscle tone that started emerging through my flesh was pretty rad. My body has definitely shifted into the look that I was going for before."

And those are just the visible results. Over time, heavy lifting routines can take a toll on your joints, and tight muscles can eventually pull your skeleton out of alignment. But with its emphasis on lengthening and stretching the body, yoga helps decompress the spine, staving off degenerative disc diseases. And with more supple joints and flexible muscles, you're much less prone to arthritis and injury. Regular yoga practice will keep you in the gym for the long haul, and give you better results from your traditional workouts—and can also build muscle and burn some serious fat all on its own.

"Try adding one or two yoga classes to your weekly training split," Kiley says, "and you'll start noticing miracles happening everywhere."

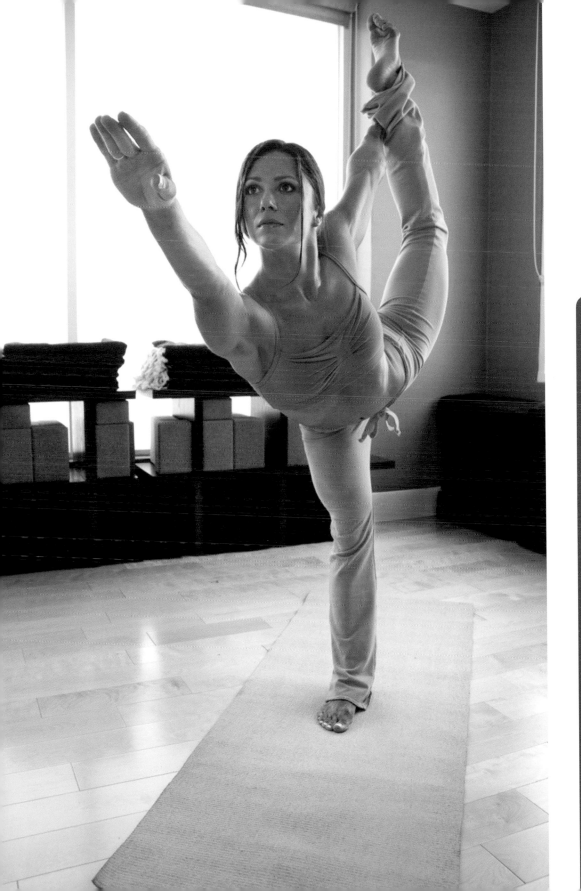

YOGA GUIDE

Which type of yoga is right for you? Here, we break down five of the most popular options to help you decide which is the best for your goals. (Note: fat-burning and muscle-building ratings are on a scale of 1–5, 5 being the highest.)

ASHTANGA VINYASA

Fat-burning rating: 5
Muscle-building rating: 5
Recommended level: Beginner to extremely advanced
This style contains a predefined series of postures that are synchronized with the breath in a dynamic flow to generate detoxifying heat in the body. Over time, an Ashtanga Vinyasa yoga practice will build the kind of impressive core strength that allows students to

DIFFICULTY RATINGS
Ariel ranks the degree of difficulty of each pose on a scale of one to five: ★★★★★ being the hardest and ★ being the easiest.

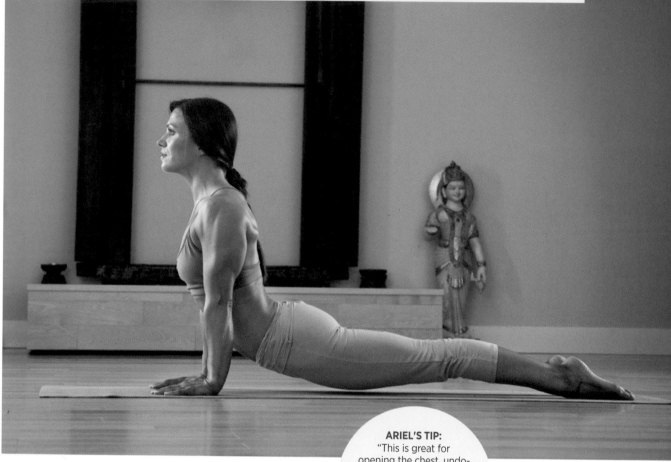

ARIEL'S TIP:
"This is great for opening the chest, undoing the chronic hunching caused by driving and sitting at computers, and also for building strength and flexibility in the legs and glutes."

UPWARD FACING DOG
★★
This is a back-bending pose, but with much of your body weight supported by the floor.

STEP BY STEP:
> Lying facedown with your legs extended, tops of feet on the floor, draw your hands underneath your elbows.
> Press your hands into the floor.
> Stack your shoulders over your wrists and press up so only your palms and the tops of your feet are on the floor.

FOR BEGINNERS: If your shoulders are too tight to perform this pose correctly, bend your elbows and lower your hips to the floor.

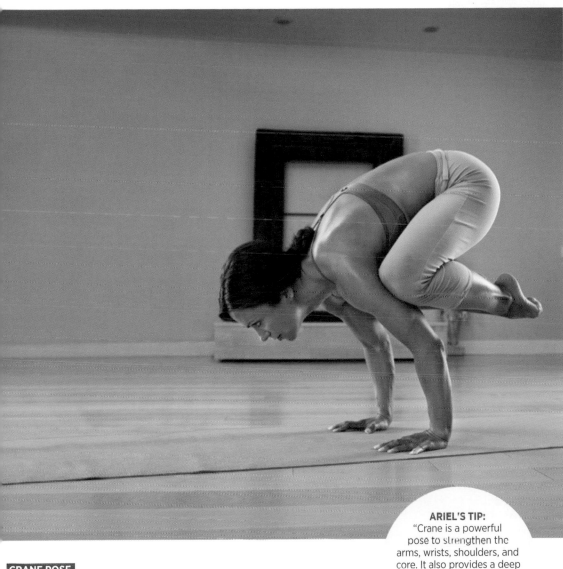

master gravity-defying poses.

BIKRAM
Fat-burning: 3
Muscle-building: 3
Recommended level: Beginner to advanced
Bikram yoga is a sequence of 26 poses performed in a room heated to at least 105 degrees Fahrenheit with 40% humidity. The goal is to sweat and detoxify the body; the elevated temperature in the room helps keep muscles limber for deeper stretches, and raises the heart rate. Therefore, Bikram yoga is more efficient at burning fat than other types.

HATHA
Fat-burning: 3
Muscle-building: 3
Recommended level: Beginner to advanced
Hatha, a Sanskrit word meaning "sun and moon," emphasizes balancing strength with flexibility. "Hatha yoga" is an umbrella phrase often used to describe all kinds of Westernized yoga classes.

IYENGAR
Fat-burning: 2.5
Muscle-building: 5
Recommended level: Beginner to intermediate, intermediate to advanced
Iyengar yoga builds muscle through the use of isometric contrac-

ARIEL'S TIP:
"Crane is a powerful pose to strengthen the arms, wrists, shoulders, and core. It also provides a deep stretch through the groin while strengthening the adductors."

CRANE POSE
★★★★★
This is an advanced, gravity-defying pose that requires significant core strength.

STEP BY STEP:
> Begin by squatting with your toes turned out and heels together, knees wide.
> Place your hands on the floor shoulder-distance apart.
> Lift your hips to snuggle your knees around the upper arms.
> Squeezing your upper arms with your knees, tighten your core to lift your navel strongly, rounding your back.
> Shift your weight forward while continuing to squeeze the upper arms with your knees.
> Float your toes off the ground, keep the toes touching, core contracted, and spine rounded as you hover.

FOR BEGINNERS: Start out perched on a block and experiment with lifting one foot at a time. Place a blanket or pillow in front of you as a "crash pad" just in case you lose your balance. Keep your tailbone as close to your heels as possible.

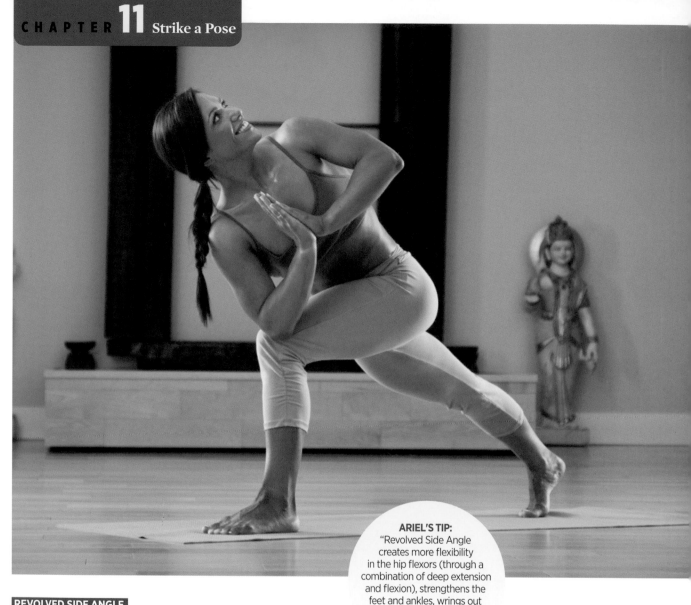

ARIEL'S TIP:
"Revolved Side Angle creates more flexibility in the hip flexors (through a combination of deep extension and flexion), strengthens the feet and ankles, wrings out (detoxifies) internal organs, and enhances balance."

REVOLVED SIDE ANGLE
★★
This is a runner's lunge, with the upper body in a powerful twist.

STEP BY STEP:
> Stand in a long lunge with your front knee over the ankle.
> Make sure your front heel is in a straight line with the back heel.
> Join palms together in front of your heart.
> Twist your torso and hook opposite elbow around outer front thigh.
> Point your other elbow toward the ceiling and look up past it.
> Press your hands together to deepen twist.

FOR BEGINNERS: Lower the back knee to rest on the floor.

tions. The focus is on achieving perfection in each pose; once in a pose, expect to stay there anywhere from three to 10 minutes or longer, making small adjustments as necessary.

POWER
Fat-burning: 5
Muscle-building: 5
Recommended level: Beginner to advanced
Power yoga is a simplified version of Ashtanga Vinyasa yoga. This version emphasizes burning fat and building muscle, and a typical class is likely to involve plenty of chaturangas—flowing through a series of motions similar to push-ups.

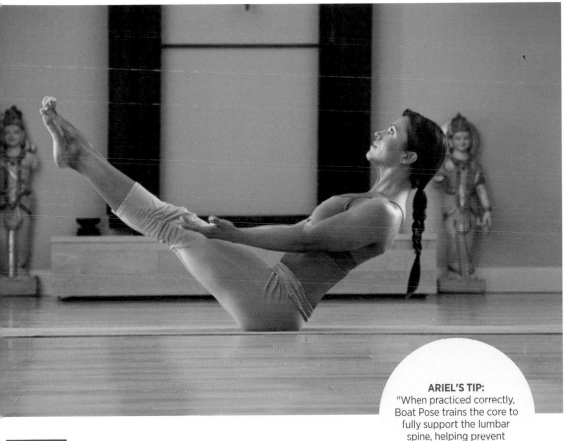

ARIEL'S TIP:
"When practiced correctly, Boat Pose trains the core to fully support the lumbar spine, helping prevent lower-back pain."

BOAT POSE
★★★
This creates a V shape between your upper and lower body.

STEP BY STEP:
> Sit on the floor with your knees bent and feet together in front of you.
> Place your hands behind your thighs and tilt your weight back until you are balancing just behind your sit bones.
> Contract your core to lift your chest and straighten the spine.
> Float your shins off the floor, then straighten your legs.
> Let go of your legs and reach your arms straight forward, palms up.

FOR BEGINNERS: Keep your hands behind your thighs and bend your knees so the shins are parallel to the floor.

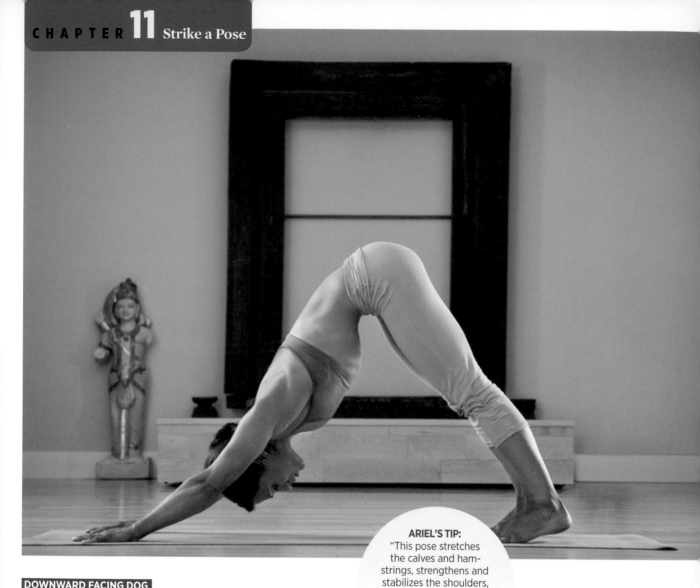

ARIEL'S TIP:
"This pose stretches the calves and hamstrings, strengthens and stabilizes the shoulders, decompresses the spine, and recirculates blood throughout the upper body."

DOWNWARD FACING DOG
★★★

This move forms a pyramid with the body, with both hands and feet on the floor and tailbone lifted high.

STEP BY STEP:
> Start on your knees with hands on the floor slightly in front of your shoulders, knees beneath hips.
> Curl your toes under, exhale and lift your hips toward the ceiling.
> Press your hands down to elongate the spine.
> Lower your heels only so much as the spine can stay straight.

FOR BEGINNERS: Bend both knees.

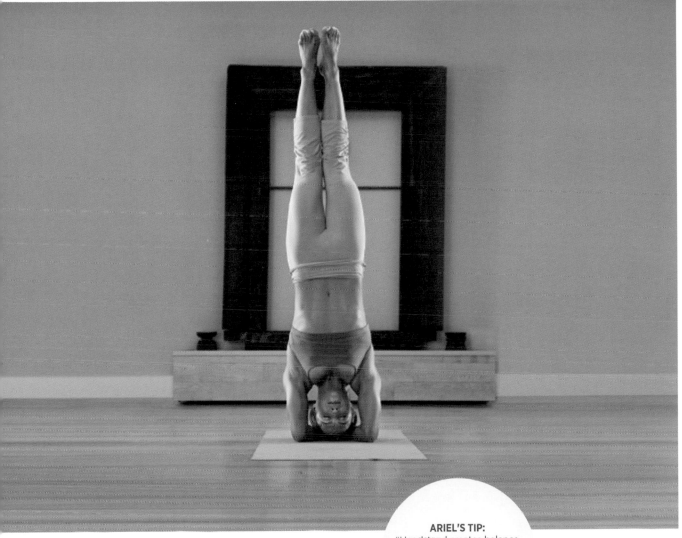

ARIEL'S TIP:
"Headstand creates balance and strength that integrates many muscles in the body—especially the arms, legs, spine, and abdominals."

HEADSTAND
★★★★★

This move is performed in steps to protect the neck. Correctly done, your head and neck will support 30% of your body weight; your core and limbs will support the rest.

STEP BY STEP:
> Starting on your knees, lace your fingers together and set your forearms on the floor shoulder-distance apart.
> Place the crown of your head on the floor, with the back of your head resting against the base of your thumbs.
> Lift your knees and walk your feet close to your body to bring your hips over your shoulders.
> Retract shoulder blades into your back to keep the spine as long as possible and protect your neck.
> Exhale and, without momentum, lift your legs to the ceiling.

FOR BEGINNERS: Practice against a wall. Bend your knees and place the soles of your feet on the wall before straightening your legs.

CHAPTER 12

Prime your body for an amazing workout and stay
injury-free with dynamic flexibility training

Stretch

Even before you drive into the gym parking lot, you pretty much know what kind of workout is waiting for you. It's going to be one of those days where every rep is a teeth-gritting effort, or it might be one of those rare times when the weights feel like they're filled with helium and your joints glide as if they've just been oiled. We've found the way to turn the former into the latter. It's called dynamic flexibility training, and it's the new-school way to prepare your body to train.

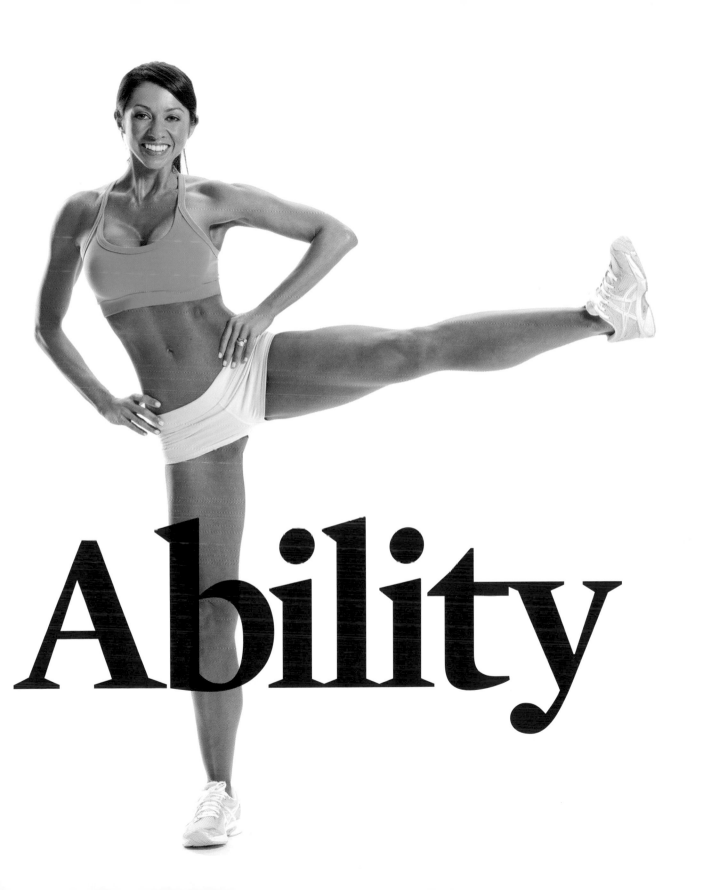

Ability

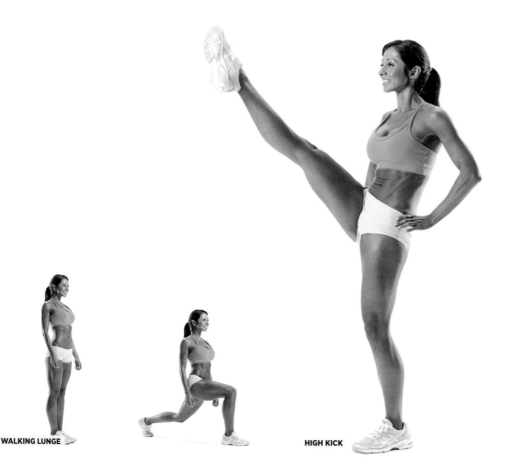

WALKING LUNGE

HIGH KICK

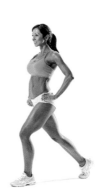

WHAT IS IT?

Dynamic flexibility training is a pre-workout routine that is designed to raise core temperature, increase joint mobility, and introduce some specificity of training to your body so your central nervous system knows what to expect when the workout begins. A dynamic flexibility routine (also referred to as a "dynamic warmup") is a series of multiplanar, explosive body-weight moves typically performed in a circuit fashion before your main workout.

Unlike static stretching, which involves holding a pose that elongates your muscles for an extended period of time, dynamic flexibility training is nearly constant motion. And unlike ballistic motions, which are designed to push your joints past their limits of mobility, dynamic movements are performed right up to the threshold of your flexibility.

WHY GO DYNAMIC?

Over the years, the separate purposes of warming up and improving flexibility have become jumbled into one effort, when in fact they are two very distinct goals that demand different approaches. The strategic use of static stretching is the tried-and-true way to improve long-term flexibility, but it's about the last thing you want to do before a hard session in the gym.

"When you do a traditional static stretch you reduce some of the stretch reflex that is in the muscle spindle. You actually lose some of that spring you get, which helps generate power," says Guillermo Escalante, Ph.D. (ABD), C.S.C.S., owner of Sport Pros training facility in Claremont, CA. "With dynamic stretching, you are warming up the muscle, but because you are not doing that long, drawn-out stretch, you maintain that explosiveness, which maintains the integrity of the stretch reflex and helps you perform better rather than worse."

HOW DO YOU PERFORM IT?

An effective dynamic warmup should take about 10 minutes. It consists of 5 to 10 moves performed in a nonstop circuit, without any external load. Start by performing five minutes of cardio on a machine that targets the body parts you plan to train. On leg day, perform the cardio on a treadmill, bike, or StepMill. If you're doing an upper-body workout, use a rower, an elliptical with handles, or a hand-bike. After the cardio, choose dynamic movements that specifically target the muscles that will be used in your workout. Perform each move for approximately 30 seconds (some will be measured in distance rather than time), and then immediately move to the next one. Begin each motion in a moderately explosive fashion, incrementally increasing the explosiveness with each rep.

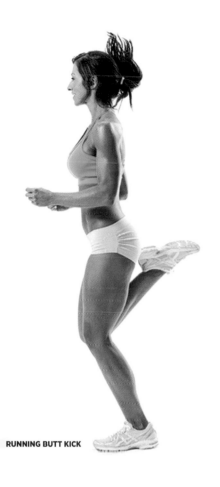

RUNNING BUTT KICK

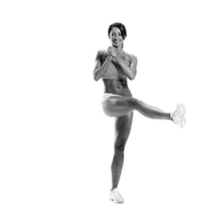

CALORIE BURNER

A dynamic warmup is meant to be strenuous. By the time you finish, you should be sweating, and your heart rate elevated, but you shouldn't be so exhausted that your workout gets compromised. It is a fine line, but it eventually pays dividends that go beyond your workout and will show in your abs and backside.

"When you perform dynamic flexibility, you burn a lot of calories because it requires you to move your butt quite a bit," Escalante says. "You are doing some sort of lunging, stepping, or swinging motion instead of just sitting down and stretching toward your toes. There's definitely a caloric-expenditure factor."

IS STATIC STRETCHING GONE FOR GOOD?

Don't fall into the trap of the swinging pendulum. Just because a new method is found to be effective doesn't mean that everything that came before it should be tossed out the window. Static stretching still has a very important place in everyone's fitness program. It's essential to improving overall flexibility for the long haul as well as recovering from injuries and mobilizing scar tissue. Perform your static stretching after your workout, when your body is still warm but you've already completed all your major lifts.

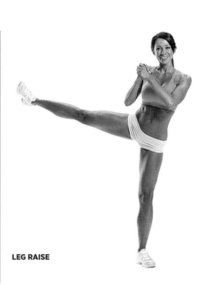

LEG RAISE

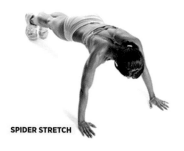

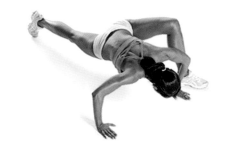

SPIDER STRETCH

Stretch It Out

Below are two sample dynamic flexibility progressions, designed to be performed before either a lower-body or an upper-body weight-training session or a track workout. Select three or four of the suggested exercises, and perform them in a circuit. Repeat the circuit two or three times, without stopping between stretches. Make sure to warm up with five minutes of low-intensity cardio.

LOWER-BODY WARMUP

Cardio	5 minutes
Lunge	20 per leg
Running Butt Kick	20 per leg
Leg Raise	20 per leg
High Kick	20 per leg
Lying Scorpion	20 per leg
Spider Stretch	30 seconds per side

UPPER-BODY WARMUP

Cardio	5 minutes
Walking Lunge	20 per leg
Hacky Sack	20 each side
Jumping Jack (not shown)	30
Side Bend	20 each side
Arm Swing	20
Arm Circle	20 each direction

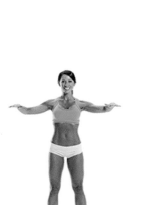

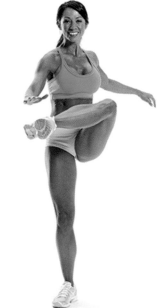

HACKY SACK

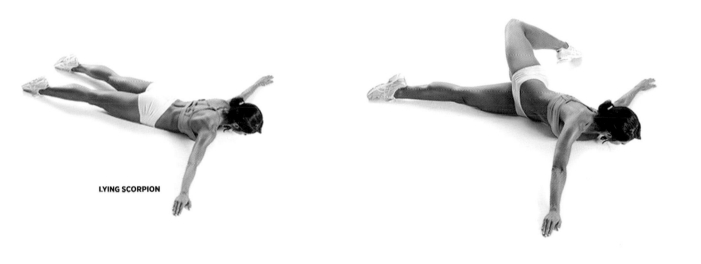

LYING SCORPION

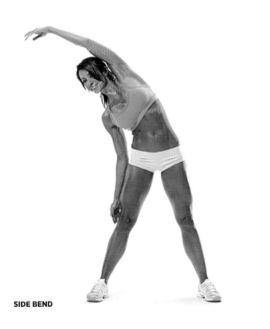

SIDE BEND

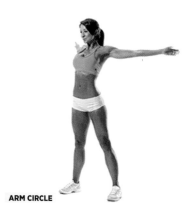

ARM CIRCLE

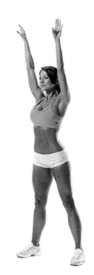

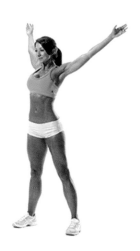

WALKING LUNGE
PRIMARY FOCUS: Hams/Glutes
SECONDARY FOCUS: Quads

> Stand with your shoulders back and down, and your feet together. Your arms can be flat at your sides or holding your hips.
> Take a big lunge forward with your right foot so that your front knee is bent 90 degrees and aligned over your ankle while your back heel is lifted off of the floor.
> Allow your back knee to come close to the floor and then push up with your back leg, transferring the weight of your body through your right heel, bringing your feet together.
> Without pausing, lunge forward with your left foot in the exact same motion and repeat.

HIGH KICK
PRIMARY FOCUS: Hamstrings
SECONDARY FOCUS: Glutes

> Stand in an athletic position with your feet shoulder-width apart and your knees slightly bent. Place your hands on your hips and step your right foot forward one-and-a-half to two feet. Your right foot should remain flat on the floor while your left heel is off the ground.
> Keeping your left knee straight and your right heel flat, kick your left leg as high as it will go. You should feel the stretch throughout your left hamstring.
> Return to the starting position just long enough to reset and kick again. Perform all the reps on one leg before switching sides.

RUNNING BUTT KICK
PRIMARY FOCUS: Quads
SECONDARY FOCUS: Hip Flexors

> Go to the aerobics room or parking lot, where you have 10–20 yards of open space ahead of you.
> Slowly run in an exaggerated manner kicking your legs up and back so that your heel strikes your glute with each kick.
> Make sure these kicks are slow and deliberate. This is not a sprint. Pump your arms to help increase the explosiveness of the kick.

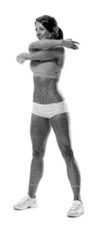

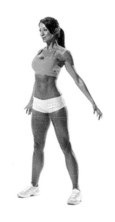

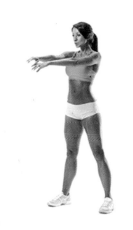

ARM SWING

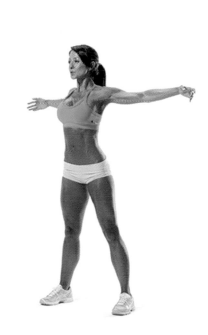

LEG RAISE
PRIMARY FOCUS: Abductors/Adductors
SECONDARY FOCUS: Glutes

> Stand in an athletic position with your feet shoulder-width apart and your knees slightly bent. Clasp your hands near your chest to help maintain your center of gravity.
> Rock your weight onto your left foot and bring your right leg across your center line and over your left toes like a pendulum. Still keeping your right leg straight, swing it out to the right side keeping your ankle flexed and your toes pointed forward the whole time.
> After it reaches its apex, allow the leg to swing freely down until it again crosses the toes of your left foot, then swing it back up in a rhythmic manner. Perform all the reps for your right leg before switching sides.

SPIDER STRETCH
PRIMARY FOCUS: Hams/Glutes
SECONDARY FOCUS: Hip Flexors

> Get on your hands and toes, in a basic pushup position. Your feet should be together, arms extended, and hands underneath your shoulders. Do not let your hips sag.
> Lower your body so there is a slight bend in your elbows. Lunge your left foot forward so it is outside your left hand.
> Hold this pose, maintaining the straight line from your right heel to your shoulders and your head in a neutral position. You should feel the stretch in the front of your right hip.

CHAPTER

13

Backside Bests

Tighten your butt fast with three workouts that will have you
ready to show off your bikini bottom

There are plenty of good reasons to get your butt in gear at the gym. And if transforming your backside has got your panties in a bunch, it's no wonder. Given the size of it (your gluteal complex, that is), finding exercises to isolate it seems nearly impossible.

With that in mind, we've sought the help of some of the top fanny bearers in the industry. Rising IFBB Pro League bikini stars Justine Munro, Nicole Nagrani, and Amanda Latona have all revealed the secrets and the workouts that help them get their backsides in tip-top shape. By following their advice, you can, too!

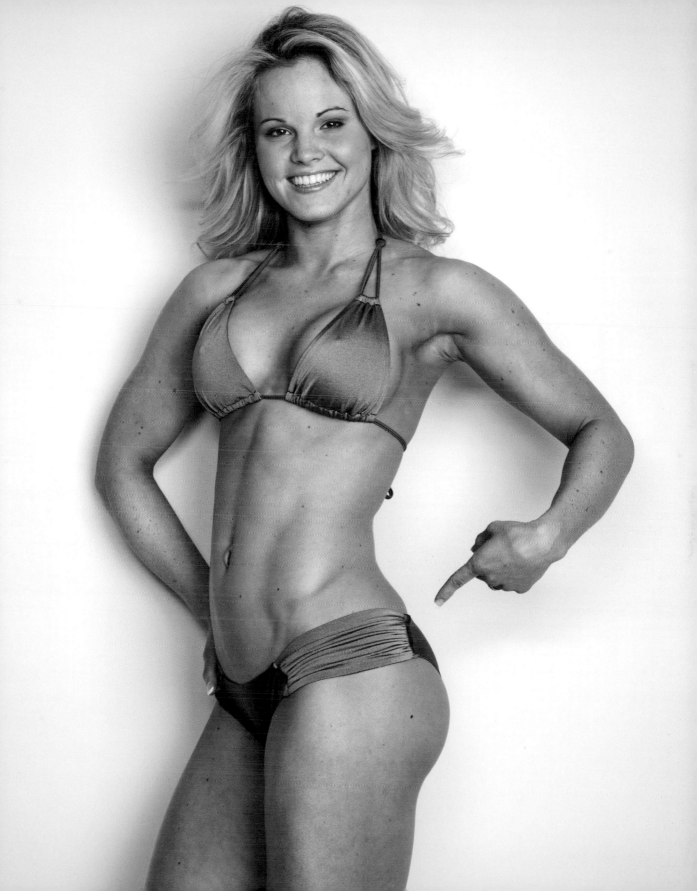

GLUTE GUIDANCE

CHOOSE MOVES WISELY

Exercises that extend the hip (move your leg backward) will better target your glutes. Glute extensions on the Butt Blaster or cable kickbacks will minimize the recruitment of nearby muscles, allowing better isolation. Lunges, squats, and step-ups are some of the best compound moves for your backside. "Lunges build up your glutes, giving them a 'lift,'" says IFBB bikini pro Nicole Nagrani. "The key is to stretch deep so you activate more of the muscle." Aim to include at least two of each type of move and vary the exercises every workout.

LIFT TO BOOST YOUR GLUTES

If you're new to exercise or haven't worked out for a few months, start by incorporating glute-specific moves in your leg workout once per week. If you've been training consistently for a few months, incorporate glute-specific moves in your leg workout and add another training day to your weekly routine that focuses only on glutes. Alternate a heavy workout (10–12 reps) with a light workout (15–20 reps).

CORRECT YOUR CARDIO

A good 30-minute dose of cardio four or five times per week will give your booty a boost—but use the machines that will kick your glutes the hardest. A study conducted at the Madonna Rehabilitation Hospital, in Nebraska, found that those who performed cardio on a treadmill, elliptical, or stair stepper got more cheek action than those who used a recumbent bike. Shake up your glutes even more by increasing the incline on the treadmill; shifting your hips back so your tush sticks out on the elliptical; and letting go of the rails on the stair stepper to force your heels down.

EAT (YES, EAT!) FOR A TIGHT BUTT

You have to cut calories to lose weight, but still stoke your body with enough carbs to fuel your training and protein to build muscle. For long-lasting energy and just the right mixture of protein, carbs, and fats to serve your goals, aim for a calorie ratio of roughly 30%, 60%, and 10%, respectively. Amanda Latona, 2010 Sacramento Pro bikini champ, suggests you stock up on lean proteins such as chicken and fish, ditch the sugars for slower-digesting carbs and more fibrous greens, and get your healthy fats from sources like almonds.

EAT MORE

To get your out-of-control booty to go down, you have to chow down. Eating more foods, in a sensible way, will help you burn more calories. "Lots of clean food is key to losing fat and creating a shapely-looking butt," says IFBB bikini pro Justine Munro. "A round booty is made of muscles, and those muscles still need fuel." For your body to receive all the nutrients it needs from food to maintain health, you need to consume a minimum of 1,600 calories per day.

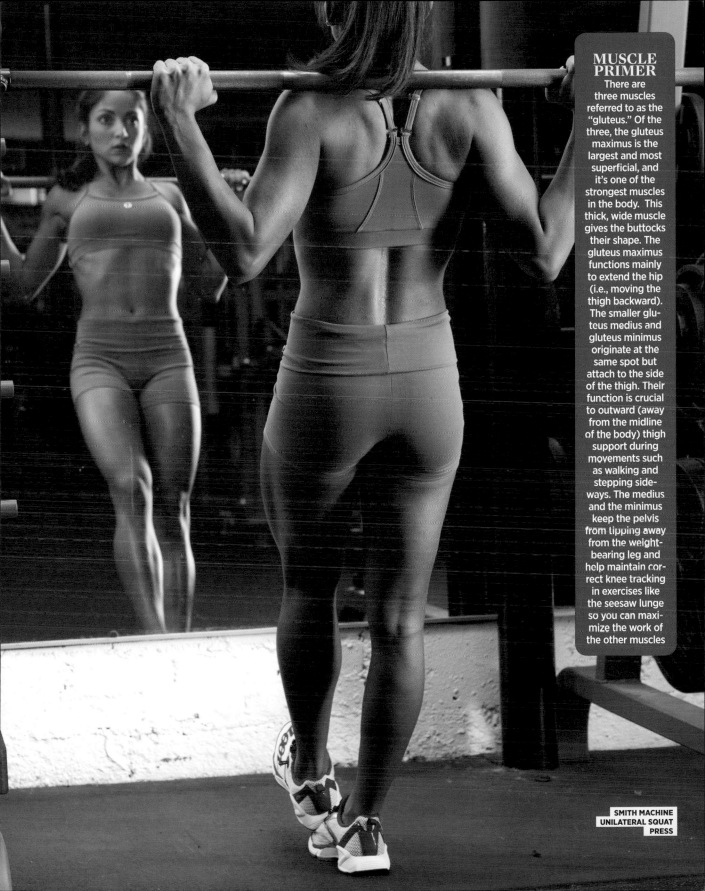

MUSCLE PRIMER

There are three muscles referred to as the "gluteus." Of the three, the gluteus maximus is the largest and most superficial, and it's one of the strongest muscles in the body. This thick, wide muscle gives the buttocks their shape. The gluteus maximus functions mainly to extend the hip (i.e., moving the thigh backward). The smaller gluteus medius and gluteus minimus originate at the same spot but attach to the side of the thigh. Their function is crucial to outward (away from the midline of the body) thigh support during movements such as walking and stepping sideways. The medius and the minimus keep the pelvis from tipping away from the weight-bearing leg and help maintain correct knee tracking in exercises like the seesaw lunge so you can maximize the work of the other muscles

SMITH MACHINE UNILATERAL SQUAT PRESS

Justine Munro's Glute Workout

	EXERCISE	SETS	REPS
1/	Unilateral Leg Press	4*	15 (each leg)
2/	Unilateral Stiff-leg Deadlift	4	15 (each leg)
3/	Pop Squat	4	25
	SUPERSET WITH		
4/	Butt Blaster	4	20
5/	Jump Lunge	4	25
	SUPERSET WITH		
6/	Good Morning	4	25

* Does not include warmup sets.
Note: Rest for 45 to 60 seconds between sets. Rest for 60 seconds between supersets.

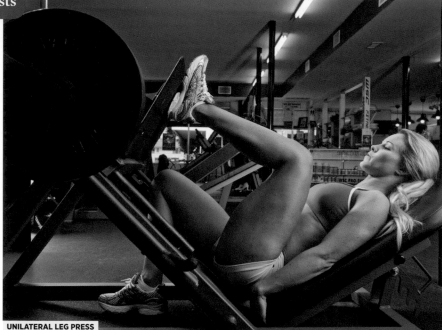

UNILATERAL LEG PRESS

1/ UNILATERAL LEG PRESS

> Position your back and shoulders squarely against the pad.
> Allow the weight to slowly push your knee toward your chest.
> Press through your heel until your leg is straight but not locked out.

2/ POP SQUAT

> Stand erect with your feet shoulder-width apart.
> Extend your arms out to your sides, or put your hands on your hips.
> Using a faster-than-usual descent, push your knees and hips down until your thighs are parallel with the floor.
> Without pausing, drive back up explosively and jump to a full standing position with feet together.
> Absorb the landing and quickly descend into a squat again.
Tip: "Don't land flatfooted. Land with your toes touching down first, then arches, then heels, so you keep your momentum going. If your knees hurt while doing this exercise, try standing in one place, then squat down and pulse up and down for the prescribed number of reps."

3/ BUTT BLASTER

> Place your foot firmly on the pad.
> Keeping a slight bend in your knee, drive your leg up and squeeze your glutes.
> Slowly return to the starting position, but don't allow the weight stack to touch down.
> Keep your back flat and your neck in line with your spine.
> Switch sides and repeat.
Tip: "Tense your glutes and hamstrings to get the full effect of each press."

4/ UNILATERAL STIFF-LEG DEADLIFT

> Stand erect with a dumbbell in each hand, palms facing your thighs.
> Keep your feet slightly narrower than shoulder-width apart.
> Bend forward from the hips, keeping your right leg planted.

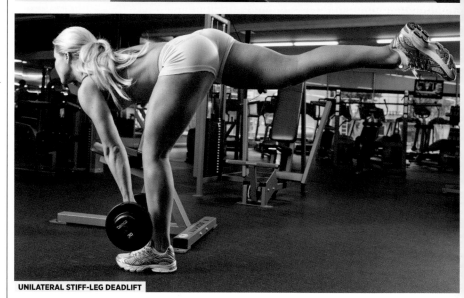

UNILATERAL STIFF-LEG DEADLIFT

> Allow your right leg to come up behind you as your torso drops.
> Push back up to standing, bringing your left foot forward to meet your right foot.
> Squeeze your glutes at the top and repeat.

5/ JUMP LUNGE

> Stand erect with one foot out in front of the other, hands on hips.
> Using a faster-than-usual descent, squat until your back knee almost touches the floor.
> Drive through the heel of your front foot, pushing explosively to get as much

height as possible.
> Quickly switch your feet before landing, then immediately descend again into a lunge.
> Repeat with opposite leg.

6/ GOOD MORNING

> Stand erect with the bar resting across your shoulders and feet shoulder-width apart.
> Keep your lower back arched and knees slightly bent.
> Bend forward at the hips until your torso is parallel to the floor.
> Return to the starting position and repeat.

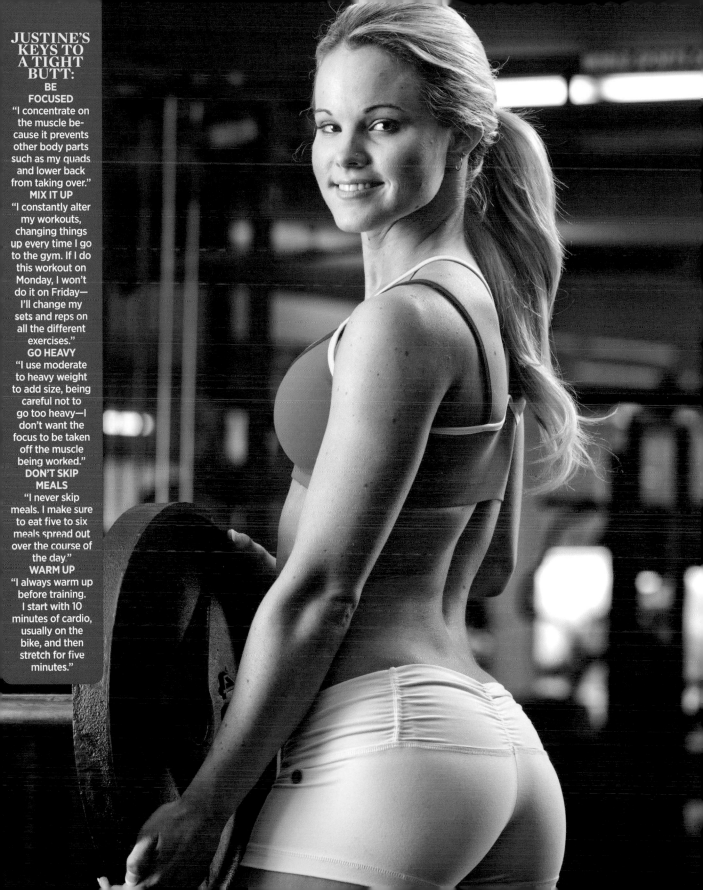

JUSTINE'S KEYS TO A TIGHT BUTT:

BE FOCUSED
"I concentrate on the muscle because it prevents other body parts such as my quads and lower back from taking over."

MIX IT UP
"I constantly alter my workouts, changing things up every time I go to the gym. If I do this workout on Monday, I won't do it on Friday— I'll change my sets and reps on all the different exercises."

GO HEAVY
"I use moderate to heavy weight to add size, being careful not to go too heavy—I don't want the focus to be taken off the muscle being worked."

DON'T SKIP MEALS
"I never skip meals. I make sure to eat five to six meals spread out over the course of the day."

WARM UP
"I always warm up before training. I start with 10 minutes of cardio, usually on the bike, and then stretch for five minutes."

NICOLE NAGRANI'S GLUTE WORKOUT

	EXERCISE	SETS	REPS
1/	Smith Machine Unilateral Squat*	5	15
	SUPERSET WITH		
2/	Dumbbell Pullthrough	5	15
3/	Dumbbell Sumo Squat	5	15
	SUPERSET WITH		
4/	Bench Step-up	5	15
5/	Standing Leg Press on Assisted Pullup Machine	5	15
	SUPERSET WITH		
6/	Unilateral Leg Press	5	15

* Does not include warmup sets.
Note: Rest for one minute between supersets.

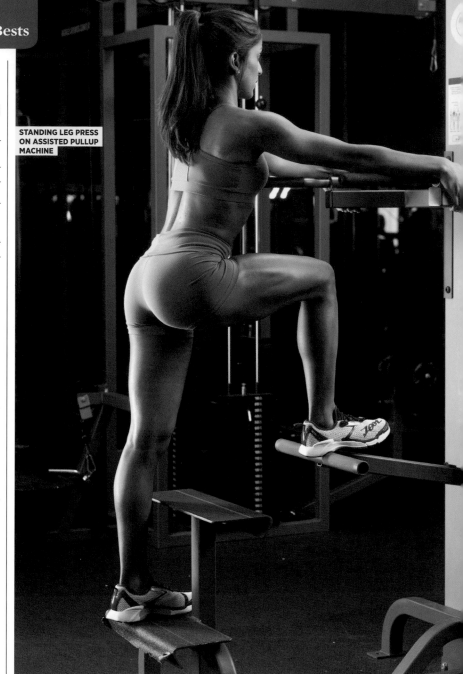

STANDING LEG PRESS ON ASSISTED PULLUP MACHINE

1/ SMITH MACHINE UNILATERAL SQUAT
> Stand erect with the bar resting across your upper traps and your feet shoulder-width apart, toes pointed forward.
> Position your feet slightly in front of the bar.
> Extend your right leg forward while keeping your left foot firmly planted on the floor.
> With your back flat, squat down until your left thigh is parallel to the floor.
> Press up through your heel, shifting your hips forward and squeezing your glutes to return to standing.
> Switch legs and repeat.

2/ DUMBBELL PULLTHROUGH
> Start with your feet a little wider than shoulder-width apart, toes pointed slightly outward.
> Hold a 20-pound dumbbell with both hands at chest level.
> With your back flat, squat down while leaning forward to push the dumbbell back between your legs.
> Press through your heels to return to standing, and raise the weight in an arc back to chest level.
> As you raise the weight, squeeze your glutes.
Tip: Focus on squeezing your glutes and your hamstrings as you pull the weight back up.

3/ DUMBBELL SUMO SQUAT
> Stand with your feet much wider than shoulder-width apart, toes pointed out.
> Hold a dumbbell in front of your thighs with both hands.
> With your upper body tilted slightly forward, bend at the knees and hips as if to sit in a chair.
> Driving up through your heels, push your hips forward and squeeze your glutes to return to upright.
Tip: "If your knees pass over your toes, your stance isn't wide enough; step out a few more inches."

4/ BENCH STEP-UP
> Stand facing a flat bench or a knee-high step.
> Place your right foot firmly on the bench and use it to lift your body weight.
> Squeeze your glutes and hams tight at the top, and touch the toe of your left foot to the bench.
> Slowly lower your weight back to the floor, leaving your right foot in place.
> Repeat for reps, then switch legs.

5/ STANDING LEG PRESS ON ASSISTED PULLUP MACHINE
> Put your right foot on the right step of the machine and your left foot on the middle of the assist platform.
> Keeping your back straight, push down on the platform until your leg is fully extended.
> Resist the platform back up until your right thigh is past parallel with the ground.
> Repeat for reps and switch sides.
Tip: "Make sure you push down through your heel, and forcefully contract your quad out."

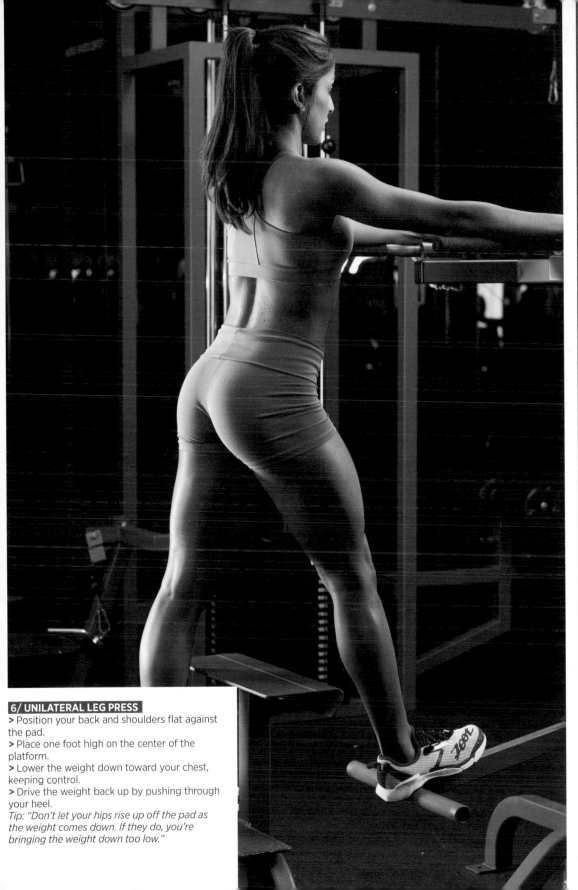

6/ UNILATERAL LEG PRESS

> Position your back and shoulders flat against the pad.

> Place one foot high on the center of the platform.

> Lower the weight down toward your chest, keeping control.

> Drive the weight back up by pushing through your heel.

Tip: "Don't let your hips rise up off the pad as the weight comes down. If they do, you're bringing the weight down too low."

NICOLE'S KEYS TO A TIGHT BUTT:

USE VARIETY

"I change things up every time I train my glutes to keep things fresh. One workout I might do dropsets, the next maybe a different rep range—I'll stick with five sets of each different exercise, usually pairing them as supersets."

WATCH FORM

"I use good form on all exercises; I keep my back straight, and head and chest up to ensure I am hitting the targeted muscle properly."

LUNGE

"I use lunges a lot in my training because they work my glutes the hardest to add size. I sometimes use them in my cardio routine, lunging instead of walking while I'm on the treadmill."

EAT CLEAN

"I always eat clean foods. I eat lots of protein, healthy fats, and complex carbs to ensure my muscles are being feed with healthy nutrients."

GO DEEP

"I go as deep as possible on all glute exercises. Maximizing muscle activation in each and every exercise is always my goal."

AMANDA LATONA'S GLUTE WORKOUT

	EXERCISE	SETS	REPS
1/	Leg Press	3*	12–15
2/	Walking Lunge	3	12–15
3/	Reverse Lunge	3	12–15
4/	Butt Blaster	3	10–15
5/	Bench Step-up	3	12–18
6/	Cable Kickback	3	12–15

Does not include warmup sets.
Note: Rest for 45 to 60 seconds between sets.

1/ LEG PRESS

> Place your feet high and slightly wider than shoulder-width apart on the sled.
> Keep your chest up and back pressed against the pad.
> Bend your knees to lower the sled, stopping before your glutes lift off the pad.
> Drive up through your heels until your legs are straight, but not locked.

Tip: "Keep your feet flat on the platform, but focus on pressing with your heels for more glute emphasis."

2/ WALKING LUNGE

> Stand erect and hold a dumbbell in each hand, palms facing your thighs.
> Step forward with one foot and drop your hips straight down by bending at both knees.
> Once your front thigh is parallel to the floor, push back up to standing.
> Step forward with the opposite foot and repeat.

3/ REVERSE LUNGE

> Stand erect with your feet about hip-width apart.
> Step back with one foot, and bend your knees and hips to descend toward the floor until your back knee almost touches.
> Push up to standing, bringing your back foot forward to meet the front.
> Step forward with the opposite foot and repeat.

Tip: "Don't let your front knee bend more than 90 degrees or move past the front of your toes."

4/ BUTT BLASTER

> Keeping a slight bend in your knee, drive your leg up and squeeze your glutes.
> Slowly return to the starting position, but don't allow the weight stack to touch.
> Keep your back flat and your neck in line with your spine.
> Switch sides and repeat.

Tip: "Tense your glutes and hamstrings to get the full effect of each press."

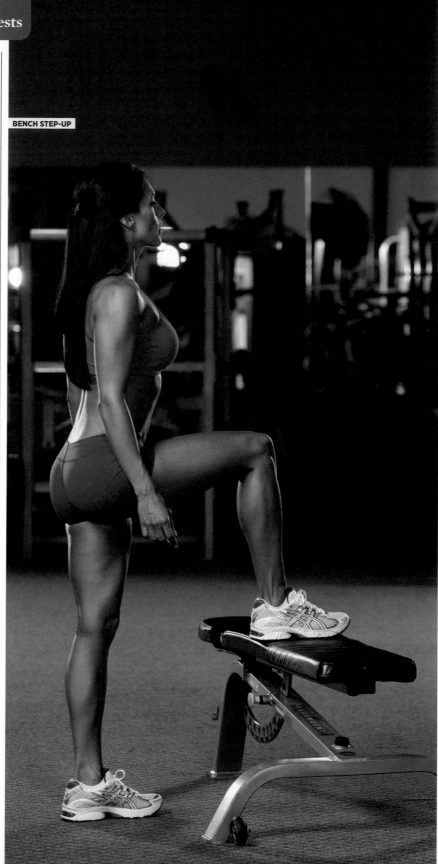

BENCH STEP-UP

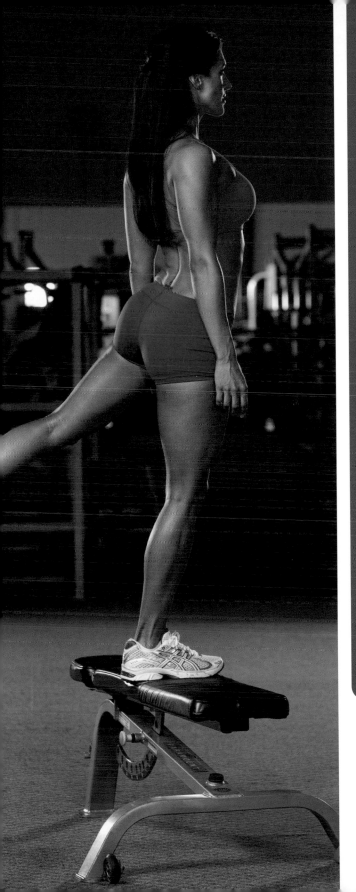

GO HEAVY

"I use heavy weight to add size, and I always keep my rep range between 12 and 15 for all three sets."

DO PLYO

"I use plyometrics to increase the intensity of my workouts. I'll do plyo drills, such as jump squats, for a maximum of 30 seconds between sets of exercises."

STEP IT UP

"I do my cardio on a stepper-type of machine after my weight training. If I use the gauntlet one day, then I'll use the stair stepper the next. If I add in a third workout, I'll replace my cardio with the stair stepper in between sets."

DRINK H$_2$O

"I always drink lots of water because it flushes toxins from the body and helps boost my metabolism."

SKIP SUGAR

"I never eat sugar; I pair my protein with slower-digesting carb sources like brown rice, yams, and fibrous green veggies."

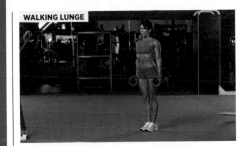

WALKING LUNGE

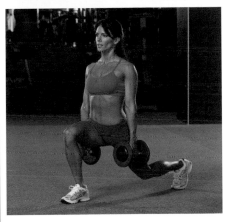

5/ BENCH STEP-UP

> Stand facing a flat bench or a knee-high step.
> Step up with your right foot, placing it firmly on the bench.
> Squeeze your glutes as you push up, pausing briefly at the top.
> Slowly lower your weight back to the floor, and repeat.

6/ CABLE KICKBACK

> Attach an ankle cuff to a low pulley cable and fasten it around your ankle.
> Stand facing the weight stack and take a step back with your nonworking foot.
> Keeping a slight bend in your working knee, drive your leg straight back.
> Slowly bring your leg forward, resisting the pull of the cable, until you reach the starting position.

CHAPTER 14

Build YOUR OWN Biceps

Take matters—along with barbells, dumbbells, and D-handles—into your own hands and get ready to show off your arms

There's nothing more eye-catching to the weight-trained eye than a pair of well-toned, well-defined biceps. Maybe that's because the arms are one of the few body parts that are often on display. It is socially acceptable, after all, to wear sleeveless dresses in a way that, say, wearing midriff-revealing garments just isn't.

But building sculpted biceps isn't always easy, and without the right training program you could be selling yourself short. So check out this comprehensive piece on everything biceps, and get ready to show off when you shed your long sleeves.

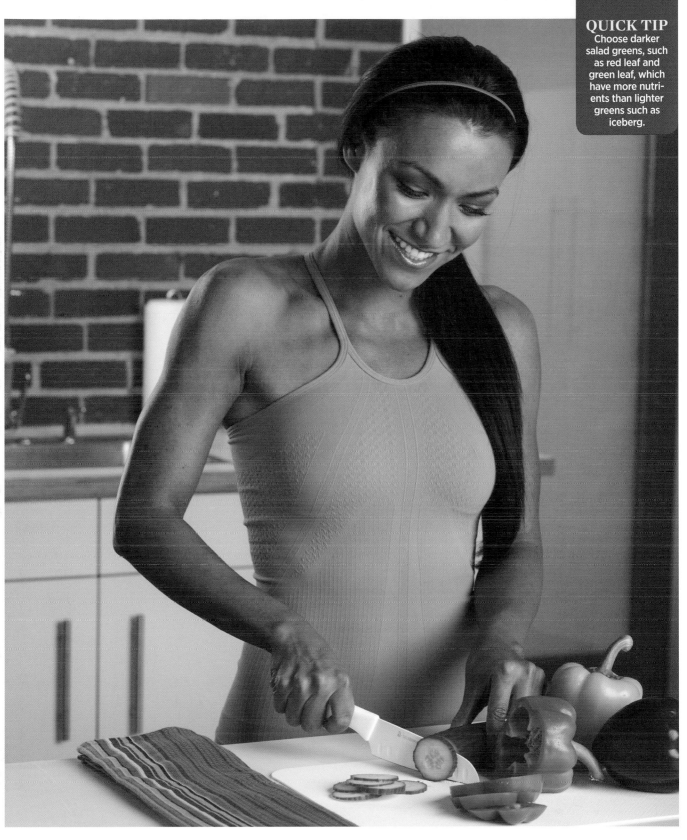

CHAPTER 17

THE Girls Guide to Supplements

Supplements can give you that extra edge to burn fat and gain lean muscle faster. Here's a list of the 15 best.

A good, hard, training regimen is the only way to get a perfectly lean body, and it releases all those endorphins that make you feel awesome afterward. But by all estimates, a sound nutritional program accounts for around 80% of your results. What those accounts don't, er, account for is the power of supplements. Add these 15 critical elements to your diet and you'll supercharge your lean muscle gains, accelerate fat loss, and improve your overall health.

SYMBOL KEY

All of these supplements have numerous benefits. Below is a symbol guide showing the primary benefits of each supplement.

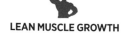 **LEAN MUSCLE GROWTH**   **FAT BURNING**   **OVERALL HEALTH**   **INCREASES STRENGTH**   **INCREASES ENERGY**

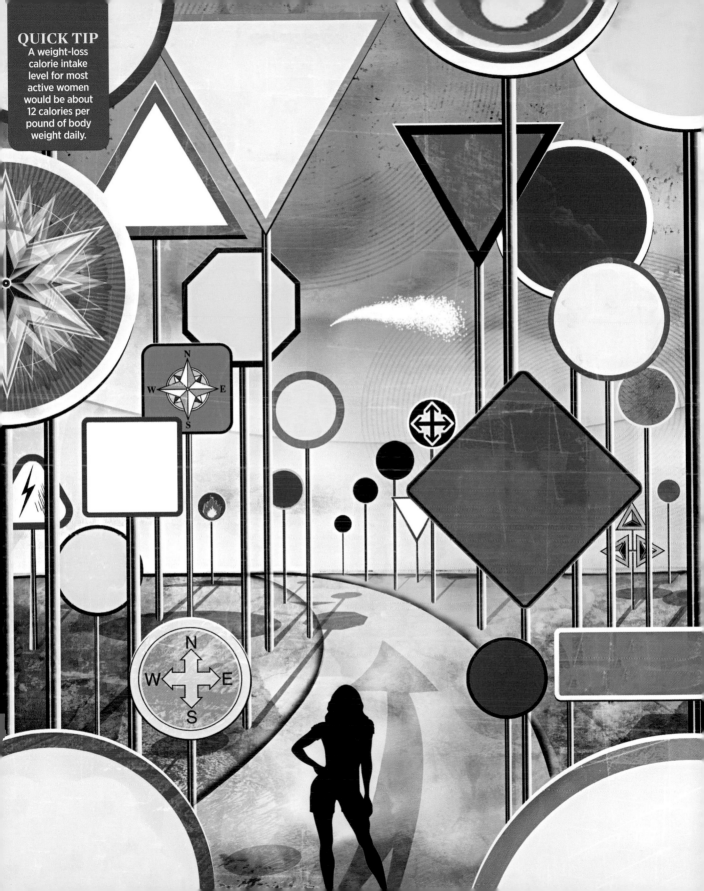

1 Whey Protein

What it is: One of milk's two proteins

What it does: Whey's primary characteristic is its digestibility. Once in the body, it breaks down quickly, sending its aminos to muscle tissue. This is beneficial because there are certain times of day (first thing in the morning, before and after workouts) when the lean, whole-food proteins we normally recommend (eggs, chicken breast, lean steak, fish) digest too slowly to be effective. But whey doesn't deliver only protein. It contains peptides (protein fragments) that have been shown to increase blood flow to muscles, which is particularly helpful before workouts, so then muscles will receive more oxygen, nutrients, and hormones right when they need them.

How to take it: Take 20 grams of whey protein (mixed in water) first thing upon waking, within 30 minutes before workouts, and within 30 minutes after training. And you can always have a scoop as a snack between meals.

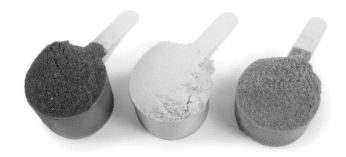

2 NO Boosters

What it is: Any number of compounds that serve to increase levels of nitric oxide in the bloodstream

What it does: NO relaxes the muscles that control blood vessels, which makes them increase in diameter, allowing more blood to flow through them and to muscles. Because blood carries oxygen and nutrients such as glucose, fat, and amino acids, more of these getting to your muscles allows for better energy production—so you can train harder for longer—and better recovery from workouts, which means bigger muscles that can be trained more often. Blood also contains a high percentage of water, which gets pushed through those wider blood vessels into muscles to create the muscle pump you experience when you train. That pump stretches the membranes of muscle cells, signaling the cells to grow bigger. In addition, NO enhances lipolysis, which is the release of fat from the body's fat cells, allowing it to be burned for fuel.

How to take it: Look for products that include ingredients such as arginine, citrulline, GPLC (glycine propionyl-L-carnitine), or pycnogenol. Take one dose of an NO-boosting supplement about 30–60 minutes before workouts.

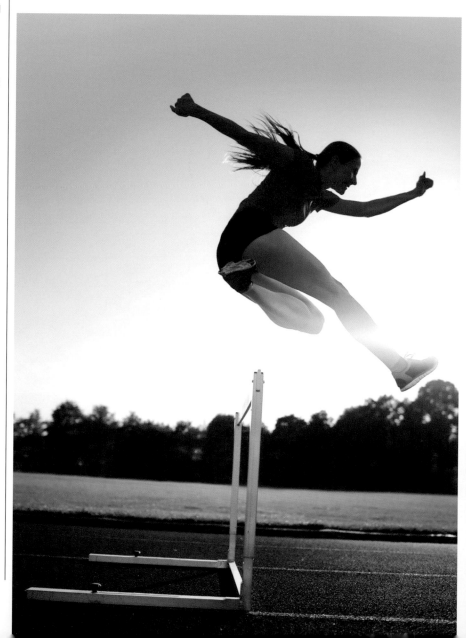

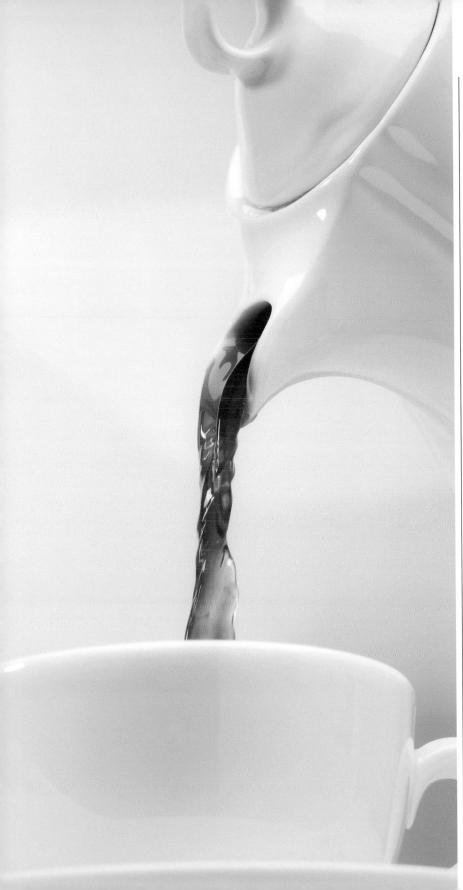

3 Caffeine

What it is: Only the world's most popular (and legal) stimulant drug

What it does: You already know it perks you up and improves focus, but it also has been found to boost muscle strength, intensity, and fat loss during workouts. And it works especially well when taken with green tea extract. Caffeine increases the amount of fat that gets released from your fat cells. Meanwhile, green tea boosts metabolic rate, which is the way the body burns fat in the bloodstream. Taking these compounds together means that more of the fat that caffeine has released will get burned up for good, allowing your fat cells to shrink away.

How to take it: Take 200–400 milligrams of caffeine two or three times per day, with one dose 30–60 minutes before workouts.

4 Fish Oil

What it is: Two essential omega-3 fatty acids, eicosapentaenoic acid (EPA) and docosahexaenoic acid (DHA)

What it does: What *doesn't* fish oil do? It reduces inflammation; reduces muscle and joint recovery; reduces risk of heart disease, diabetes, and cancers; and, a biggie, it also has been found to turn on genes that stimulate fat burning and turn off genes that increase fat storage.

How to take it: Take 2 grams of fish oil three times daily, with breakfast, lunch, and dinner.

5 Casein Protein

What it is: The other of milk's two proteins

What it does: Though they come from the same place, whey and casein couldn't be more different. Casein is extremely slow to digest, which means it provides a steady stream of aminos over a span of several hours. That makes it ideal for certain time periods, like right before bed, when your body is about to go without food for seven to eight hours. In fact, one study performed by the Weider Research Group found that when subjects took casein protein before bed, they gained more muscle than those who took casein in the morning. Another study found that when subjects consumed a mix of whey and casein after workouts, they had improved muscle growth as compared with subjects who took just whey.

How to take it: Take 20 grams of casein right before bed. Also consider combining 10 grams of casein with 10 grams of whey in your post-workout shake.

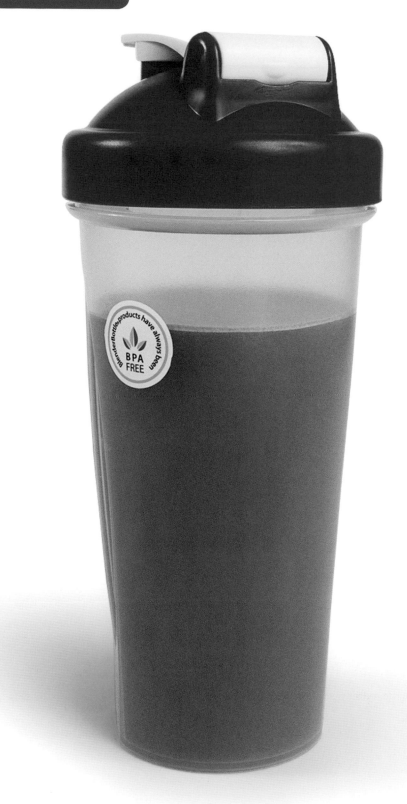

6 BCAAs

What it is: Three aminos (isoleucine, leucine, and valine) that share a branched molecular structure

What it does: The unique structure of BCAAs gives them certain unique properties, all of which have physique benefits. BCAAs can increase the length of your workouts—they can be burned as fuel by muscle tissue and they actually blunt fatigue in the brain. The BCAAs are also intimately involved in the creation of new muscle tissue, both as the building blocks and as the builder. Leucine, in particular, promotes protein synthesis, which is the process by which muscle grows. BCAAs also boost growth-hormone levels, reduce cortisol, and increase levels of insulin, the anabolic hormone that's critical to replenishing muscle tissue with nutrients after workouts.

How to take it: Take 5–10 grams of BCAAs with pre-workout and post-workout shakes.

7 Creatine

What it is: An amino-acid-like compound that occurs naturally in muscle tissue

What it does: Creatine's most basic function is to help muscles create fast energy during exercise. Taking supplemental creatine increases the amount of energy the body has to draw upon, increasing endurance and strength. The compound also draws water into muscle cells, increasing their size and causing a stretch that can yield permanent growth.

How to take it: Take 2–5 grams of creatine (depending on the form you use) before and after workouts with pre- and post-workout shakes.

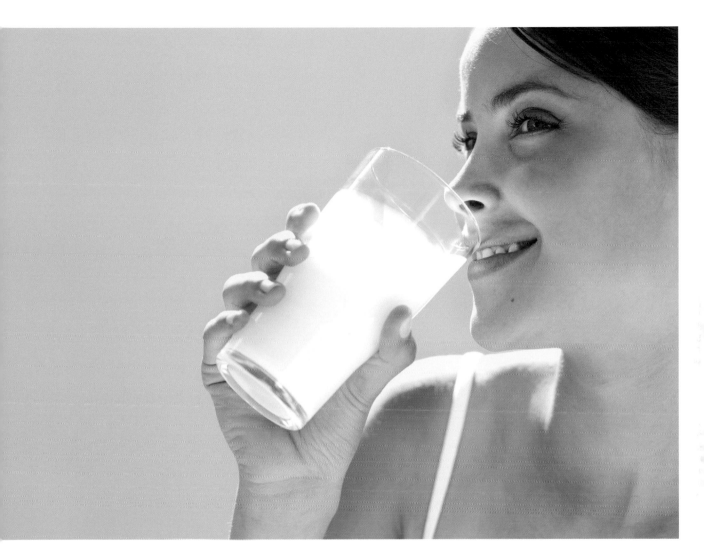

8 Beta-alanine

What it is: A nonessential amino acid
What it does: When beta-alanine meets another amino acid, histidine, a beautiful thing happens: They get together and form a compound called carnosine. Carnosine has been shown to improve muscle size, strength, and endurance and increase fat loss. Since the amount of carnosine the body can produce is directly dependent on how much beta-alanine is present, it makes sense to supplement with beta-alanine.
How to take it: Take 1–3 grams of beta-alanine immediately before and immediately after workouts.

9 CLA

What it is: A healthy fat that just happens to be an omega-6 fatty acid
What it does: Although other omega-6 fats are not so healthy, primarily because Americans tend to get too much of them in their diet, CLA is different. Numerous studies confirm that it enhances fat loss while simultaneously boosting muscle growth and strength. It works by two mechanisms: decreasing the amount of fat that is stored in fat cells and boosting metabolism. It also appears to burn more fat during sleep, thereby sparing muscle tissue.
How to take it: Take about 2 grams of CLA three times daily, with breakfast, lunch, and dinner.

10 Calcium

What it is: An essential mineral
What it does: Just about everyone knows that calcium is intrinsically linked to bone health, but did you know that it's also required for muscle contraction? Without adequate calcium, muscles won't contract properly. And research shows that this unassuming mineral can also help spur fat loss, particularly the fat around your midsection. This may be because calcium decreases the amount of dietary fat that's absorbed by the intestines and suppresses a hormone called calcitriol, which is responsible for fat production and reducing fat burning.
How to take it: Take 500–600 milligrams of calcium twice a day.

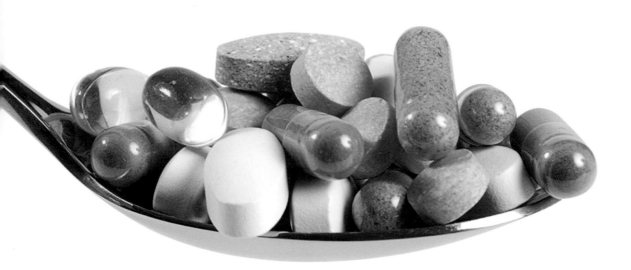

11 Vitamin D

What it is: The sunshine vitamin

What it does: New research keeps coming, all of it demonstrating D's ample health benefits, from protecting against cancer and other diseases to improving bone integrity, which it does by assisting with calcium absorption. Vitamin D is also associated with greater muscle strength—interacting with receptors on muscle fibers to activate genes that increase muscle strength and growth. As a plus, D can aid fat loss, especially when taken in conjunction with calcium.

How to take it: Take about 2,000 international units (IUs) of vitamin D twice a day at the same time you take calcium.

12 Green Tea Extract

What it is: Active ingredients in green tea, particularly the polyphenol epigallocatechin gallate

What it does: EGCG blocks an enzyme that normally breaks down norepinephrine, a neurotransmitter/hormone related to adrenaline that increases metabolic rate and fat burning, keeping norepinephrine levels higher. Green tea extract also has been found to enhance muscle recovery after intense workouts, as well as aid joint recovery.

How to take it: Take about 500 milligrams of green tea extract standardized for EGCG three times daily before meals, with one dose about 30–60 minutes before workouts.

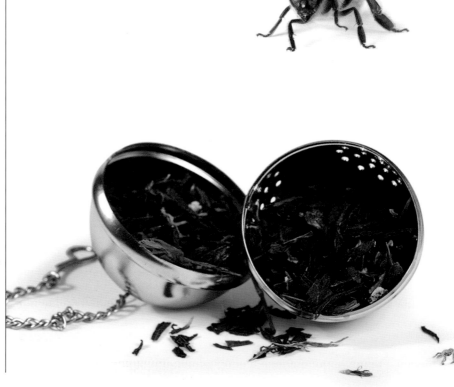

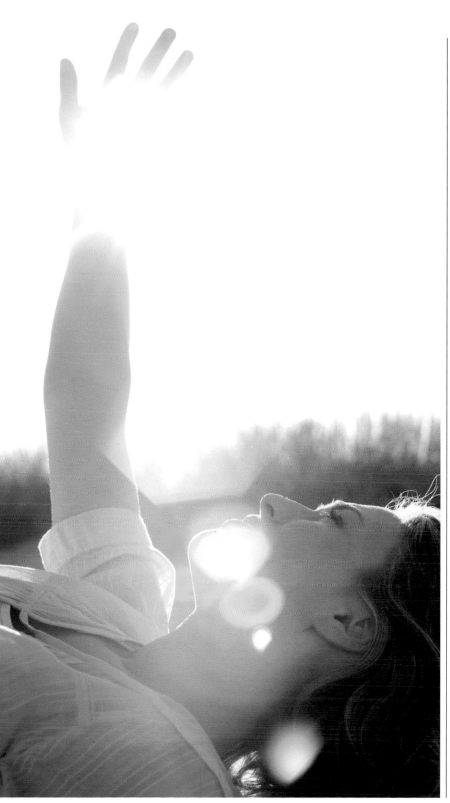

13 B Complex 100

What it is: A series of essential vitamins
What it does: Think of it this way: B makes you buzz. The suite of B vitamins are critically involved in helping your body derive energy from the nutrients you eat and helping get oxygen to muscle tissue. Feeling rundown and lacking energy? It's likely because you're deficient in B vitamins, a common trait of hard-training individuals. Certain B vitamins have additional benefits—riboflavin can help the body digest and use the protein you're eating to make sure you're building muscle properly; and folic acid, in addition to being essential to fetal health, is involved in NO production in the body.
How to take it: Look for a B complex 100, which will provide 100 milligrams of most of the B vitamins, including thiamin (B1), riboflavin (B2), niacin (B3), pantothenic acid (B5), and pyridoxine (B6), as well as at least 100 micrograms of cobalamin (B12), folic acid (B9), and biotin (B7).

14 Vitamin C

What it is: An essential vitamin
What it does: At the first sign of a tickle in your throat you probably start mainlining the C. That's good, because the vitamin has been shown to boost immune function. Vitamin C is a powerful antioxidant that is also involved in the synthesis of hormones, amino acids, and collagen; and on top of all that, it destroys free radicals, created from exercise and other stressors, that break down nitric oxide. Sparing NO from free-radical damage means you'll have higher NO levels, and higher NO levels lead to increases in muscle endurance, a reduction in fatigue, and an increase in lean muscle growth and strength.
How to take it: Take 1,000 milligrams twice a day with meals.

15 Multivitamin

What it is: A blend of adequate amounts of major micronutrients
What it does: Put simply, a multivitamin/multimineral complex fills in all the nutritional gaps in your diet. And, although we suggest you supplement separately with calcium and vitamins B, C, and D, you should still take a standard multi. It will help eliminate the possibility of deficiencies in some of the other vitamins and minerals that can result from reduced food variety or calorie intake (read: dieting) and increased vitamin loss from exercise. Being deficient in many of these micronutrients can lead to low energy levels and restrict muscle growth, strength gains, and fat loss.
How to take it: Look for a multi that provides a minimum of 100% of the daily value of C, D, E, and most of the B-complex vitamins and at least 100% of zinc, copper, and chromium. Take it once per day with a meal, such as breakfast.

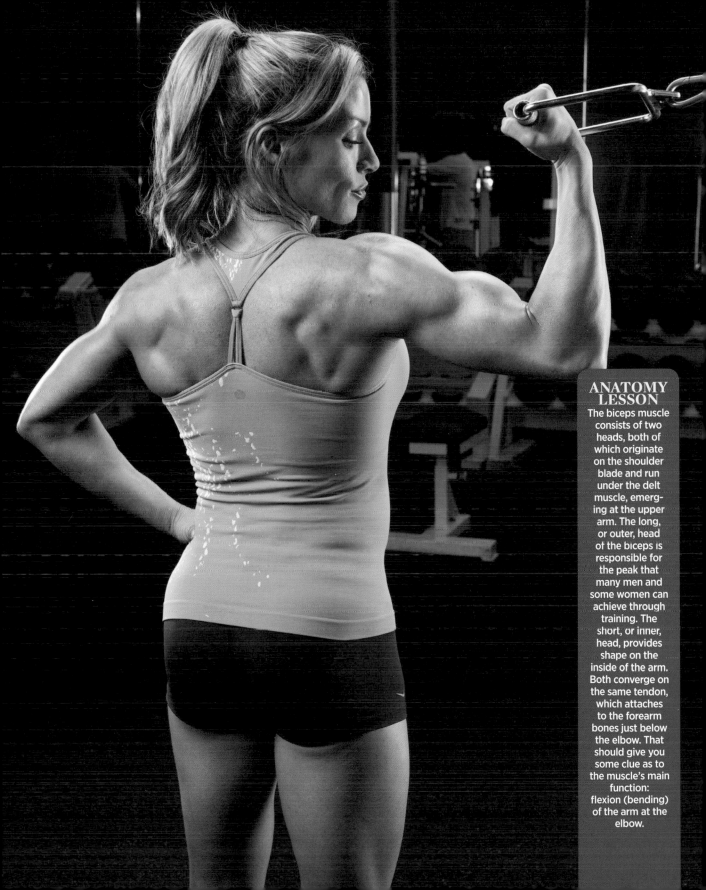

ANATOMY LESSON

The biceps muscle consists of two heads, both of which originate on the shoulder blade and run under the delt muscle, emerging at the upper arm. The long, or outer, head of the biceps is responsible for the peak that many men and some women can achieve through training. The short, or inner, head, provides shape on the inside of the arm. Both converge on the same tendon, which attaches to the forearm bones just below the elbow. That should give you some clue as to the muscle's main function: flexion (bending) of the arm at the elbow.

KNOW YOUR BI'S
In order to build an incredible set of arms, you need to know more than simply how to curl a dumbbell. Here, we answer some of the more common questions concerning how to properly train biceps.

HOW OFTEN SHOULD I TRAIN BICEPS?
Most people train biceps once a week. However, sticking with the same split for the rest of your life is a sure way to watch your progress sputter, if not come to a screeching halt altogether. Since the biceps are in your crosshairs right now, consider bumping up your training frequency by adding another biceps day to your split.

SHOULD I TRAIN BICEPS ALONE?
The larger the amount of muscle that you target with each workout, the better the growth-hormone (GH) response. Since the arm muscles are too small to cause a real boost in GH levels, your body relies particularly heavily on growth hormone to assist with gains in muscle size and strength and to reduce body fat. So it's fine to train biceps with triceps, but only if you're also training a major muscle group on that same day.

WHAT'S THE BEST NUMBER OF TOTAL SETS WHEN TRAINING BICEPS?
Between 6 and 12 sets per workout, depending on how many exercises you choose to do. You could do the typical two to four exercises with three sets each or you could choose to do fewer exercises for more total sets per exercise.

WHAT'S THE BEST REP RANGE?
Exercise science tells us that the best rep range for building muscle is 8–12 reps. That goes for every muscle group. However, that doesn't mean that you want to do 8–12 reps every single workout. Use 8–12 reps as your base rep range, and occasionally mix it up by going as low as 5–6 with heavier weights and as high as 15–20 reps with lighter weight.

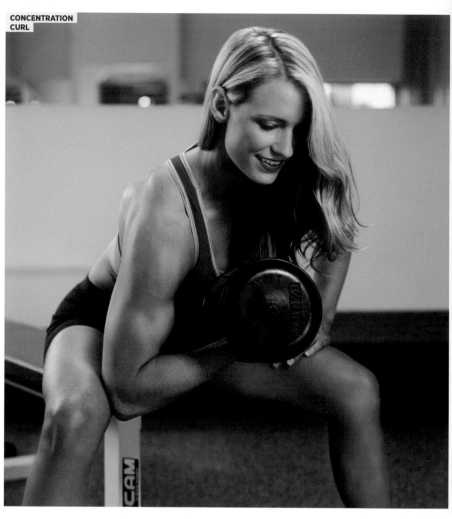

CONCENTRATION CURL

CHOOSE YOUR WEAPON
Although the curl is the main exercise to use for training biceps, there are many attachments to choose from when you are using cables. Here's a primer on what to use and why to use them.

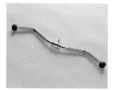

EZ-CURL BAR
Allows you to have more of a neutral grip. The more neutral the grip, the more involvement you get from the long head of the biceps, which is the one that gives you the best peak. It's called "EZ" because it's easier on the wrists.

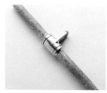

STRAIGHT BAR
Allows you to use a closer grip, which puts more stress on the outer head of the biceps.

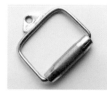

D-HANDLE
Essentially a dumbbell for cable exercise. Cables provide constant tension on the muscle, whereas, with free weights, there are certain areas in the range of motion when you're no longer putting stress on the muscle.

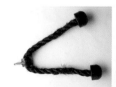

ROPE
Use this to get a truly neutral grip, putting the most emphasis on the outer head of the biceps.

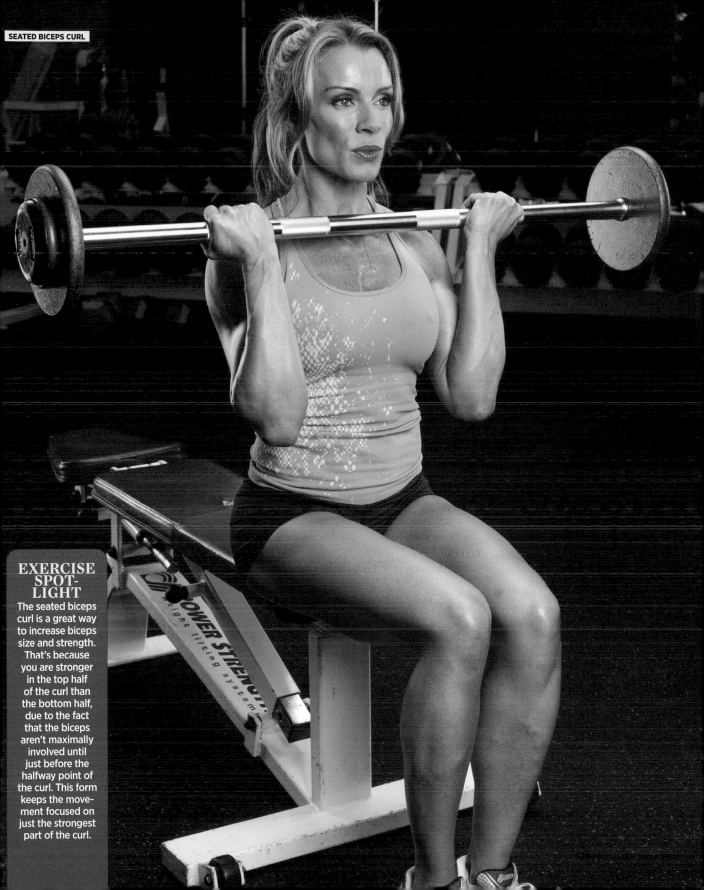

SEATED BICEPS CURL

GROUP 1: BUILDERS

These exercises allow you to hit both heads of the biceps evenly. Select one or two exercises from this list to do first in your workout:

Standing Barbell Curl
Seated Barbell Curl
Standing EZ-bar Curl
Preacher Curl
Standing Dumbbell Curl
Seated Dumbbell Curl

SAMPLE BICEPS WORKOUT

EXERCISE	SETS	REPS
Barbell Curl	3	8–12
Preacher Curl	3	8–12
Prone Incline Curl	3	8–12
Hammer Curl	3	8–12

PREACHER CURL

> Sit at a preacher curl bench and grab an EZ-curl bar, palms facing up, with your hands on the inside curves of the bar.
> Keep your shoulders pulled back and your chest up.
> Curl the weight up to your shoulders, squeezing for a two-count at the top.
> Lower the weight to the starting position and repeat.

STANDING BARBELL CURL

> Stand holding a straight bar, palms facing forward, with your hands slightly wider than shoulder width apart.
> Keep your back straight and chest up.
> Curl the weight up to your shoulders and squeeze at the top of the movement.
> Lower the weight slowly and repeat.

SEATED BARBELL CURL

> Sit on a bench with your feet flat on the floor. Rest the barbell on your thighs.
> Hold the barbell with an underhand grip, ensuring your hands are shoulder-width apart.
> Keeping your back straight, curl the weight up by bringing your hands toward your shoulders.
> Lower the weight back to the start position and repeat for reps.

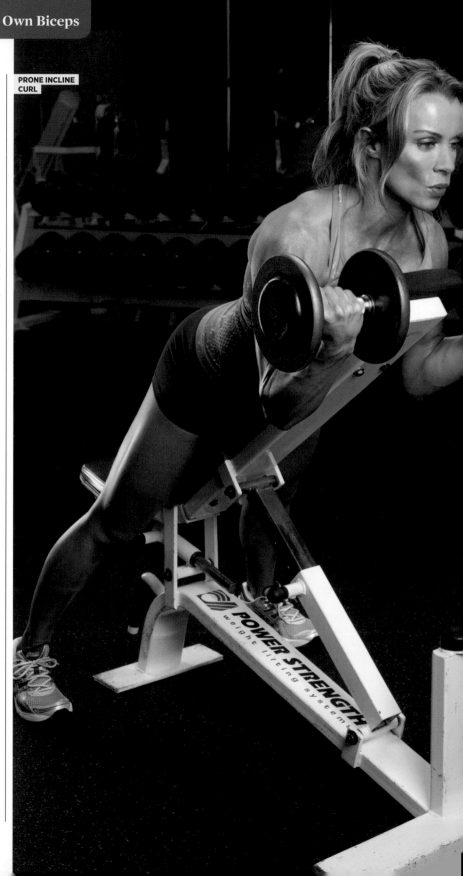

PRONE INCLINE CURL

BUMP UP THE INTENSITY

Intensity training techniques can be valuable tools. Here are a few to try. **For dumbbell curls and machine exercises:** Try adding a dropset. On the last set of each exercise, hit muscle failure, then reduce the weight by 20–30% and continue lifting until you hit failure again. **For barbell moves:** Do the rest-pause technique. On the last set of the exercise, reach muscle failure, but instead of reducing weight, reduce the rest period. Take only 10–15 seconds before eking out a few more reps. **Also try supersets:** For biceps, those would be called compound sets, or two exercises for the same muscle group performed back to back. Pick any two exercises, ideally those in which you don't risk losing your station if you're at the gym. Do one set of the first exercise, rest and then go immediately into the other exercise, alternating until you've completed all sets for both exercises. Compound sets are a great way to get better results in less time, stimulating muscle growth while also bumping up fat loss.

STANDING BARBELL CURL

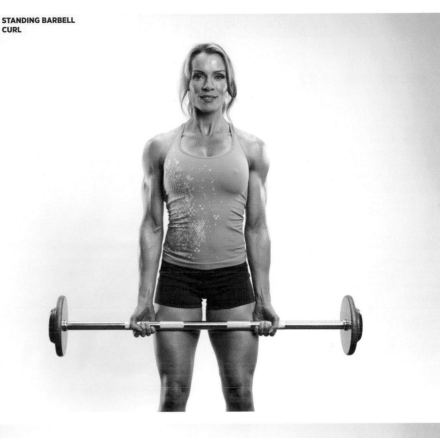

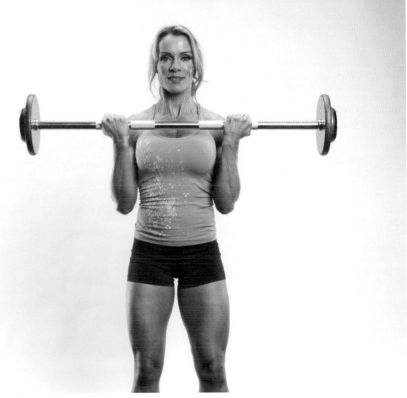

GROUP 2: SHAPERS

These exercises limit the ability to cheat and/or focus more on one head than the other. Select two exercises from this list, making sure one of them focuses on the outer head:

(OVERALL FOCUS)
Incline Dumbbell Curl
Prone Incline Dumbbell Curl
Concentration Curl
EZ-bar Cable Curl
Straight Bar Cable Curl
Cable Single-arm Curl
High Cable Curl

(OUTER-HEAD FOCUS)
Behind-the-back Cable Curl
Hammer Curl (dumbbell or rope)
Reverse-grip Barbell Curl
Reverse-grip Cable Curl

PRONE INCLINE DUMBBELL CURL

> Set an adjustable bench to a 45-degree angle.
> Lie facedown on the bench with your chest pressed firmly against the pad and your head above the top of the seatback.
> Letting your arms hang on either side of the bench, hold a set of dumbbells with an underhand grip.
> Raise the dumbbells up toward your shoulders.
> Squeeze, then slowly lower the dumbbells back to the start position.

HIGH CABLE CURL

> Stand in the middle of a cable pulley station, holding a D-grip handle in an underhand grip in each hand. Your arms should be about parallel to the floor.
> Keeping your upper arms stationary, curl the handles toward your shoulders.
> Hold for a moment at the top, then return slowly to the start position.

BEHIND-THE-BACK CABLE CURL

> Attach a D-grip handle to a low pulley and hold with an underhand grip.
> Stand slightly to the left and in front of the pulley with your legs in a staggered stance.
> Extend your arm back behind your body at about a 45-degree angle.
> Curl the weight toward your shoulder, keeping your upper arm locked in the 45-degree position.
> Return slowly to the start position.

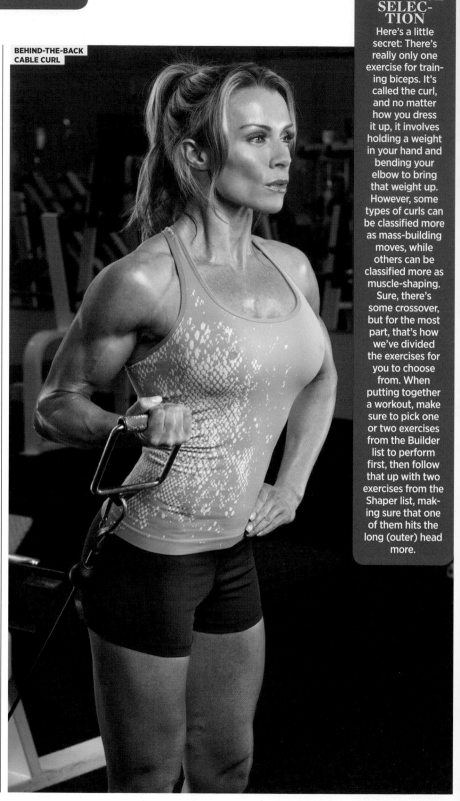

BEHIND-THE-BACK CABLE CURL

Here's a little secret: There's really only one exercise for training biceps. It's called the curl, and no matter how you dress it up, it involves holding a weight in your hand and bending your elbow to bring that weight up. However, some types of curls can be classified more as mass-building moves, while others can be classified more as muscle-shaping. Sure, there's some crossover, but for the most part, that's how we've divided the exercises for you to choose from. When putting together a workout, make sure to pick one or two exercises from the Builder list to perform first, then follow that up with two exercises from the Shaper list, making sure that one of them hits the long (outer) head more.

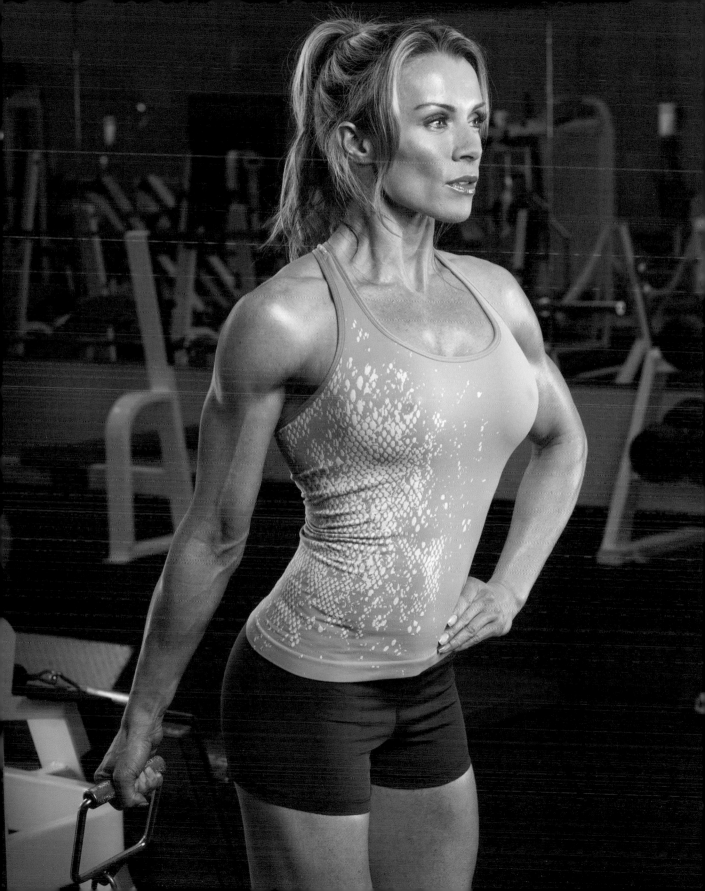

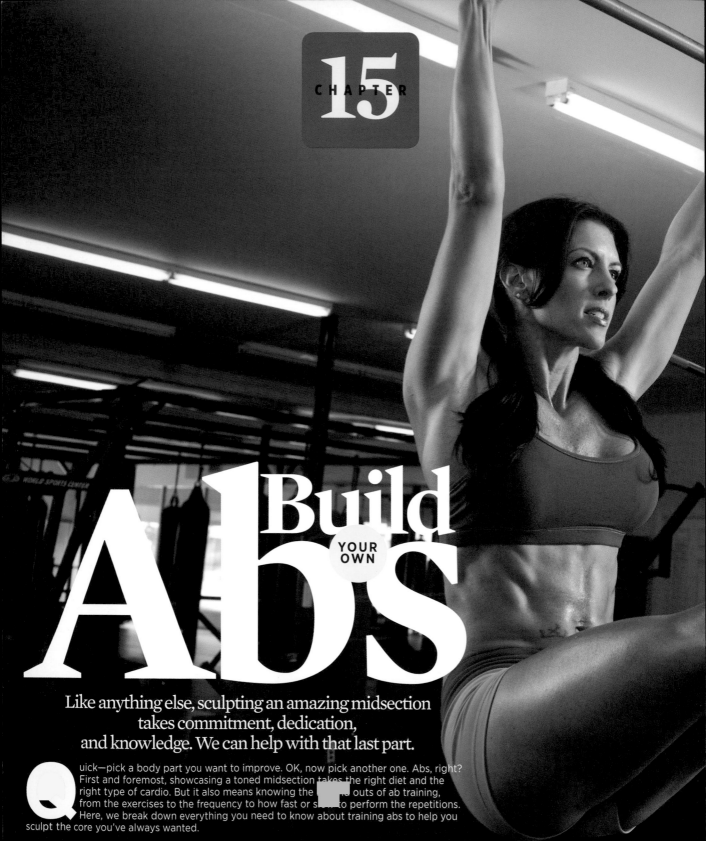

Build
YOUR OWN
Abs
1

Like anything else, sculpting an amazing midsection
takes commitment, dedication,
and knowledge. We can help with that last part.

Quick—pick a body part you want to improve. OK, now pick another one. Abs, right?
First and foremost, showcasing a toned midsection takes the right diet and the
right type of cardio. But it also means knowing the ins and outs of ab training,
from the exercises to the frequency to how fast or slow to perform the repetitions.
Here, we break down everything you need to know about training abs to help you
sculpt the core you've always wanted.

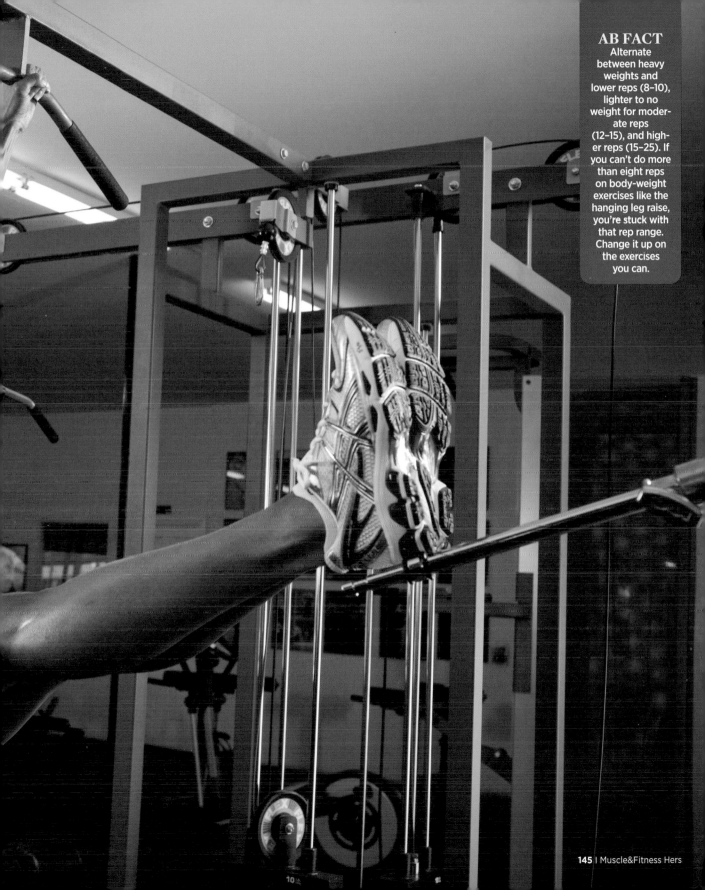

THE WORKOUT

Putting together an ab program is very simple, as long as you remember one thing: There's a strict order to the exercises. When picking from the moves below, always choose lower-ab exercises first, then upper, then obliques and finally overall core. This is the principle of priority training, where you focus on the weaker areas by doing the hardest exercises first. You can substitute any exercise that works the same abdominal region when you put together your own workout.

GROUP 1: LOWER ABS

Recommended Exercises:
Exercise Ball Reverse Crunch
Hanging Knee Raise
Hanging Leg Raise
Hip Thrust
Reverse Crunch
Exercise Ball Roll-in

SAMPLE AB WORKOUT

AB REGION	EXERCISE	SETS/REPS
Lower Abs	Hanging Leg Raise	2–3/failure
Upper Abs	Cable Crunch	2–3/10–15
Obliques	Russian Twist	2–3/15–20
Core	Cable Woodchop	2–3/15–20

HANGING LEG RAISE

> Grasp a pullup bar with an overhand grip and let your body hang from it.
> Keeping your legs straight, lift them as far past parallel to the floor as you can, rounding your back at the top.
> Pause for one second at the top before returning to the start.
Note: For a less-advanced version, use the vertical bench designed for this exercise.

HIP THRUST

> Lie faceup on the floor with your hips at a 90-degree angle and legs pointed up.
> Contract your abs, and lift your hips and glutes off the floor.
> Hold the peak-contracted position for a moment before returning to the start.

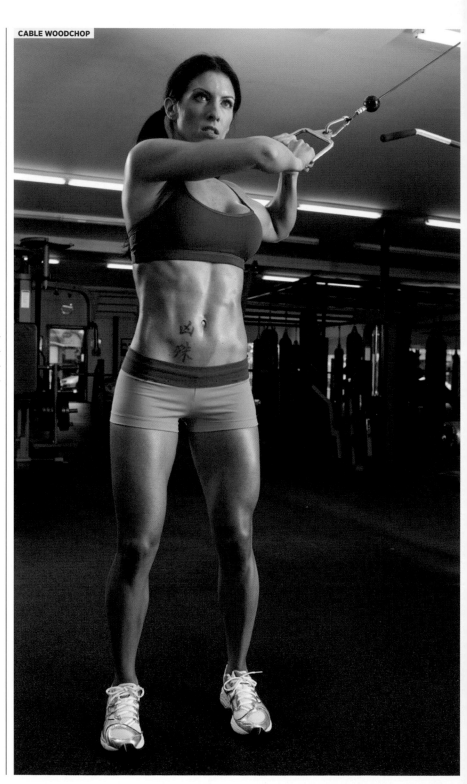

CABLE WOODCHOP

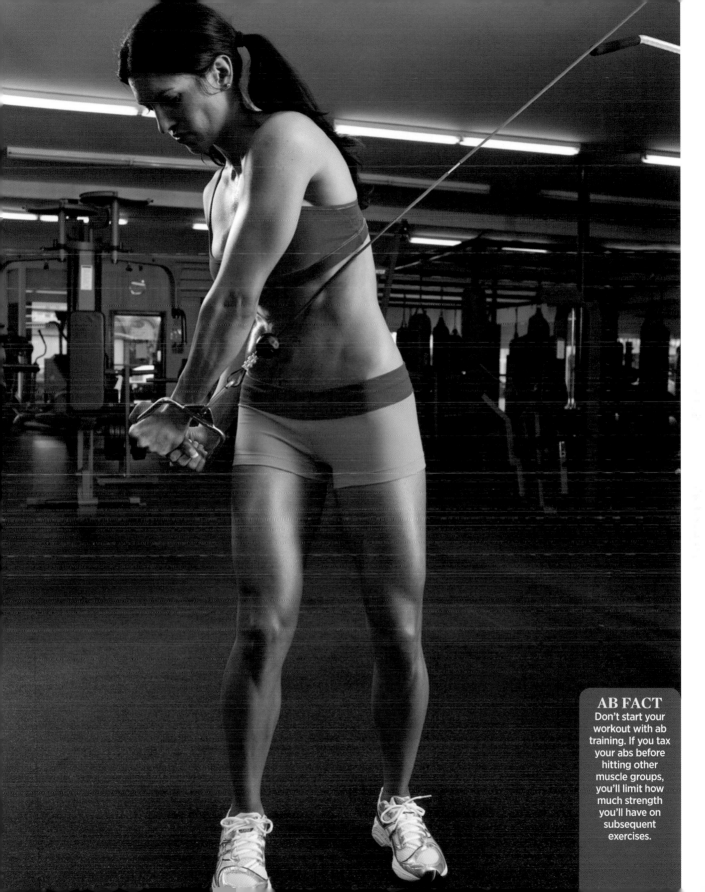

GROUP 2: UPPER ABS

Recommended Exercises:
Cable Crunch
Decline Crunch
Dumbbell V-sit
Exercise-ball Crunch
Straight-leg Crunch
V-up
Weighted Crunch

CABLE CRUNCH

> Attach a rope to a high-pulley cable station and kneel facing the weight stack.
> Grasp the rope with both hands, bend your elbows and pull it down to about ear level.
> Bend at the waist and, keeping your back parallel to the floor and arms locked, curl your elbows to your knees.
> Contract your abs before returning to the start.

WEIGHTED CRUNCH

> Lie faceup on the floor, knees bent and feet flat on the floor. Hold a weight plate at your chest with both hands.
> Keeping your eyes focused on the ceiling, lift your shoulders off the floor.
> Contract your abs and return to the start position.

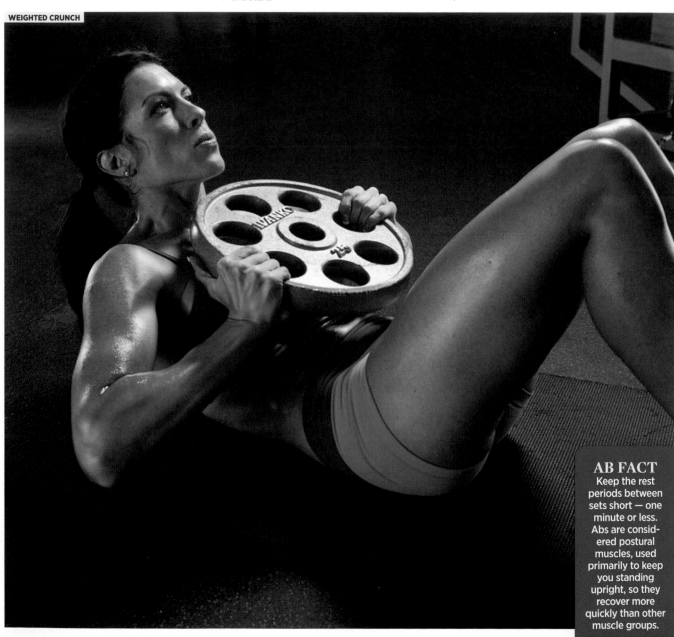

WEIGHTED CRUNCH

AB FACT
Keep the rest periods between sets short — one minute or less. Abs are considered postural muscles, used primarily to keep you standing upright, so they recover more quickly than other muscle groups.

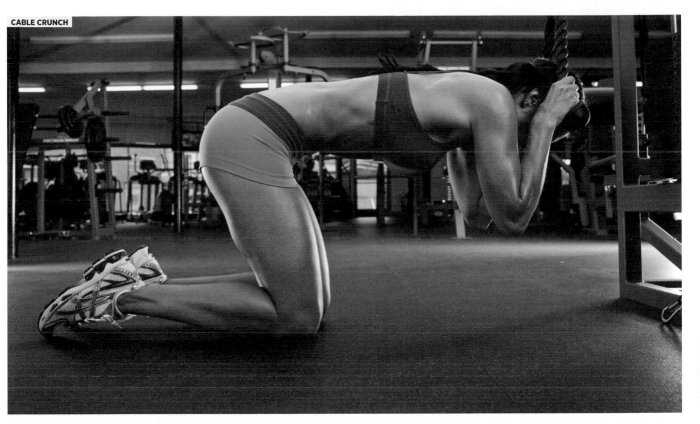

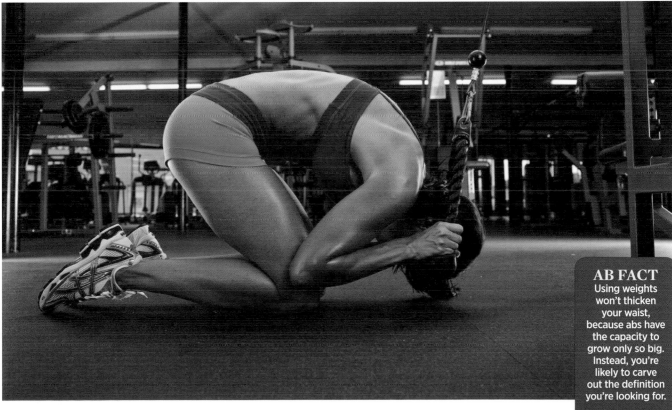

AB FACT
Using weights won't thicken your waist, because abs have the capacity to grow only so big. Instead, you're likely to carve out the definition you're looking for.

GROUP 3: OBLIQUES

Recommended Exercises:
Crossover Crunch
Oblique Crunch
Reaching Crossover Crunch
Russian Twist
Standing Dumbbell Oblique Crunch
Standing Oblique Cable Crunch
Exercise Ball Roll-in to the Side

RUSSIAN TWIST

> Sit on a decline situp bench and lean back so your abs are engaged.
> Grasp a dumbbell with both hands using a neutral grip, and extend your arms to hold it directly in front of you.
> Keeping your elbows locked and your back flat, rotate your torso to the left until your arms are roughly parallel to the floor.
> Pause for a moment, then return to the start position.
> Repeat movement to the right; that's one rep.

EXERCISE BALL ROLL-IN TO THE SIDE

> Start in a pushup position with your shins atop an exercise ball.
> Keep your legs together as you bend your knees and draw them toward your right elbow, rolling the ball forward as you do so.
> Pause, then extend your legs to return to the start. Roll the ball toward your left elbow to complete one rep.

GROUP 4: CORE

Recommended Exercises:
Cable Woodchop
Dumbbell Woodchop
Exercise Ball Pass
Exercise Ball Roll-out
Lying Leg Raise
Plank
Scissor Kick

PLANK

> Get into pushup position with your forearms on the floor.
> Only your forearms and toes should support your body. Hold the position to failure.
> Tense your core to keep your back flat.

CABLE WOODCHOP

> Attach a D-handle to a high-pulley cable station. Stand with your left side an arm's length away from the weight stack.
> Grasp the handle with both hands and start with it above your left shoulder as if you're holding a baseball bat.
> Pull the handle all the way across your body to your right hip, then pause and hold for one count.
> Repeat for reps, then switch sides.

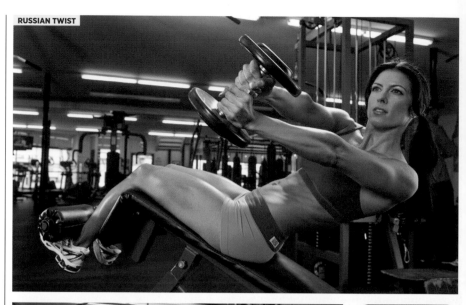

RUSSIAN TWIST

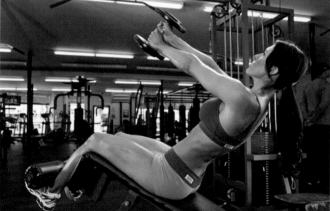

AB FACT
Just like any other muscle, abs must be broken down before they grow. To tax the muscle, you must provide what's called sufficient overload. For certain exercises, you may be able to do too many reps to be effective. That's when you need to add weight.

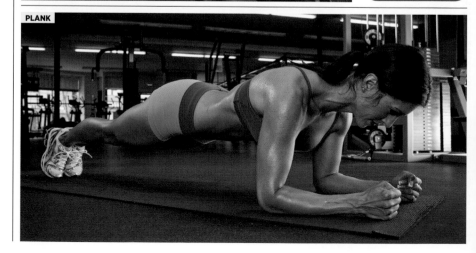

PLANK

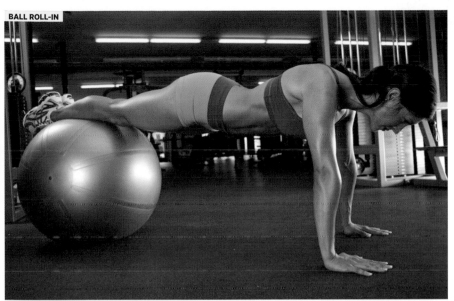

BALL ROLL-IN

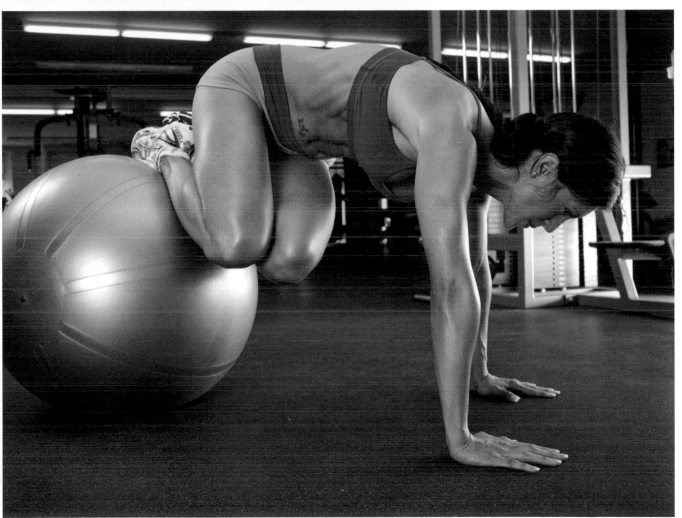

CHAPTER **16**

Nutrition
101

M&F *Hers* ultimate guide to eating right for the body you want

We don't want to burst your bubble, but a good, consistent training program alone won't get you even halfway to the body you want. Of course it's entirely necessary, and without one you won't reach your goals, but anyone who has been there and done that will tell you that the single most important factor in building the body you want is a proper nutrition plan.

We've enlisted the help of one of the best in the business—Muscle & Fitness *Hers* Senior Science Editor Jim Stoppani, Ph.D.—in compiling this comprehensive nutrition guide. Get going and get ready for your best body ever!

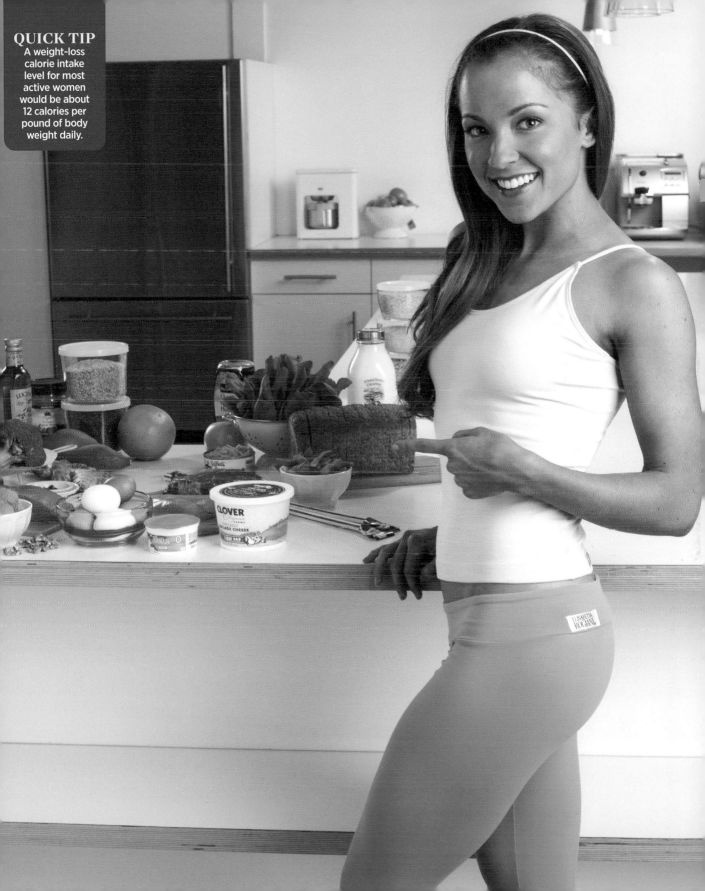

QUICK TIP
A weight-loss calorie intake level for most active women would be about 12 calories per pound of body weight daily.

Nutrition Q&A

EVERYTHING YOU EVER WANTED TO KNOW ABOUT NUTRITION, BUT WERE AFRAID TO ASK

1 If weight loss (and maintenance) really comes down to the matter of calories in versus calories out, can I reach my goal by staying under a certain amount of calories per day?
True, the most important factor for weight loss is burning more calories than you eat. But to ensure you're burning off body fat and not muscle—and to build muscle while burning body fat—your macronutrient intake becomes critical. Since muscle is composed of protein, it makes sense that you need ample amounts of protein. So when trying to drop body fat, you don't want to lower protein intake.

We now know that eating fat does not lead to fat gain, especially when you eat the right kinds—namely, essential fats like the omega-3 and monounstaurated fats. In fact, these fats actually encourage fat loss.

Unlike protein and fat, which are essential, there are no essential carbs. That's because your body can convert protein and fat into carbs. So to lose fat you should start by reducing carb intake. This method also helps to keep insulin levels low and steady, which allows for greater fat burning and less fat gain.

2 What combination of macronutrients should a healthy, active woman shoot for on a daily basis?
Typically we suggest about 1 to 1.5 grams (g) of protein, about 1g of carbs or less, and about 0.25 to 0.5g of fat per pound of body weight. That comes out to about 11 to 15 calories per pound of body weight.

3 Aside from protein, carbs, and fat, what should I be looking at on nutrition labels as far as what to eat and what to avoid?
Most of the food you eat should be fresh, unpackaged food that doesn't necessarily have a nutrition label on it—fish, chicken, steak, eggs, veggies, and fruit. This—along with your supplements—is where your micronutrients, such as vitamins and minerals, will be coming from. With packaged foods, focus on the major macros. Fiber is part of the carb macro, so the more fiber the better. And check that the sugar content is less than half the total carbs. Also be sure that there are zero trans fats, as well as nothing labeled as hydrogenated or partially hydrogentated—code words for trans fats.

4 If weight loss is predominantly about calories in versus calories out, isn't it better to skip meals if I'm not hungry?
Not really, as that can put your body in starvation mode, which slows your metabolism down and causes you to store more fat when you do eat.

5 What are the pros and cons of low-carb diets?
A lot of people complain they have no energy when eating low carb and have difficulty working out. This is true during the first couple of weeks of being on a low-carb diet. That's because in those who have been eating higher carbs, their bodies have adapted to burning carbs as a primary fuel source. When those ample carbs are suddenly gone, the body first struggles to burn adequate amounts of fat for fuel. However, after a few weeks of sticking with a low-carb diet, the body adapts by increasing the enzymes involved in burning fat, and becomes more efficient at burning fat for fuel.

6 Can I stay on a low-carb diet forever?
One problem with low-carb and low-calorie diets is that if you stay on them for too long, your leptin levels will drop. Since leptin keeps your metabolic rate up and your hunger down, lower levels of it mean that your metabolic rate also drops and your hunger rises. To prevent this, you need a high-carb, higher-calorie day about once per week.

7 Can a low-carb diet be maintained year-round, even after I've reached my goal?
There really is no reason to go back to a high-carb diet for prolonged periods. However, those on a very low-carb plan (less than 0.5g per pound) should have a high-carb day (2g or more per pound) about once per week. That's because, as stated previously, when you follow a very low-carb and low-calorie diet, your levels of the hormone leptin can start to decline. This lowers the metabolic rate and increases hunger. A day of high carbs helps raise leptin levels back up to keep your metabolism high and hunger low.

8 What are the best and worst sources of carbs?
Obviously, you want to focus on slow-digesting carbs at most meals—oatmeal, sweet potatoes, whole grains, and some fruit. One really problematic carb is fructose, which is found in fruit and in products using high-fructose corn syrup. Fructose is a sugar the body doesn't use well. The majority of fructose we consume gets converted to glucose in the body, mainly in the liver. But when there are ample glucose stores, the liver can also convert fructose into fat. So it's hard to predict whether that piece of fruit is going to be stored as glycogen or converted into fat.

OMEGA-3 FATTY ACIDS can be found in fish such as salmon, tuna, and halibut; some plants; and nut oils.

THE GLYCEMIC INDEX

The glycemic index (GI) ranks carbohydrates according to their effect on blood sugar levels. Low GI foods are burned steadily throughout the day to give you a constant supply of energy. High GI foods are readily transported to fat cells if you don't burn them off quickly. Choosing low GI carbs—the ones that produce only small fluctuations in blood glucose and insulin levels—is the secret to long-term health, reducing your risk of heart disease and diabetes, and is the key to sustainable weight loss. *Hers* recommends high GI foods only after training to spike insulin levels in order to spark lean muscle growth.

GI CHART
Foods in the low category usually have GI values of 55 or less; in the medium category, a GI value of 56–69; and in the high category, a GI of 70 or more.

Food	GI	Food	GI
Broccoli	15	White rice	64
Grapefruit	25	Table sugar (sucrose)	65
Apple	38		
Whole-grain bread	50	White bread	71
Sweet potato	54	Watermelon	72
Oatmeal	58	Rice cakes (white)	78
Pizza, cheese	60	Jelly beans	80
Spaghetti	61	White potato (baked)	85

CARBS DEFINED

A predominant energy source for your body, carbohydrates are found in a wide range of foods, such as pasta, grains, fruits, and veggies. During digestion, carbohydrate molecules are absorbed into the bloodstream and shuttled to individual cells. There, glucose—the most common form of carbohydrate—is transformed into glycogen for later use or used directly for energy. Once the body's glycogen stores are full, any extra carbohydrate is synthesized into fat.

MACRO-NUTRI-ENTS

Nutrients that the body uses in relatively large amounts—proteins, carbohydrates, and fats. This is as opposed to micronutrients, such as vitamins and minerals, which the body requires in smaller amounts.

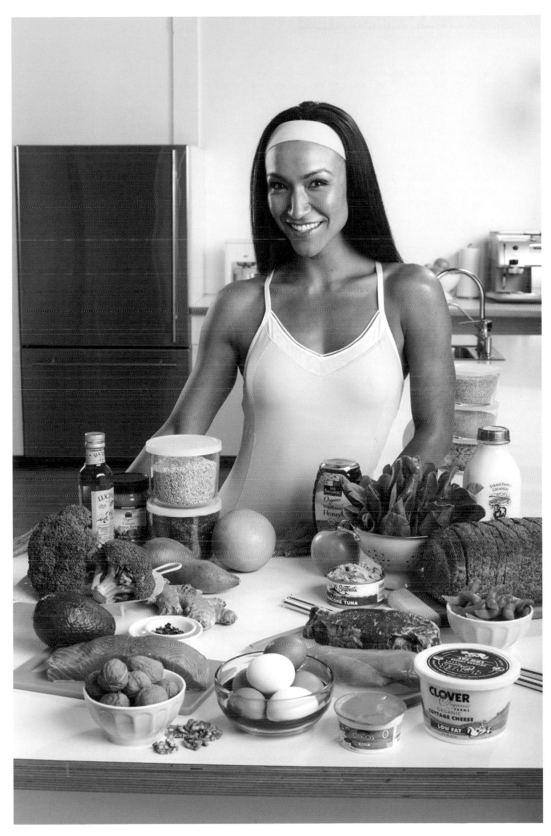

9 Should carbohydrate intake be tapered throughout the day?
Yes, most women should taper carbs, because insulin sensitivity is lower later in the day. That means that you have to release more insulin for the same amount of carbs—and since insulin inhibits fat burning, that can be bad. If you train later in the evening, you don't need to curb your intake of carbs around workouts, since they will be used to fuel the workout and recovery and won't be stored as body fat.

10 Should I avoid dairy when trying to get lean?
Not necessarily. Dairy—especially organic dairy—is not only a very high-quality protein source that is rich in glutamine, but it is a good source of conjugated linoleic acid and omega-3 fats. (For more on this, see "The 15 Best Lean-Muscle Building Foods" near the end of this chapter.) Whey protein and casein protein powders come from dairy. You simply can't get a better protein source around workouts, so why avoid them?

11 Will eating fat make me fat?
Not if you are eating the right kind of fats. Fat is an energy source, just as carbs and protein are. But fats also perform important functions in the body. They are used to make up cell membranes like those encasing muscle cells. The essential fats—the omega-3s and -6s—are used in the body to make critical chemical messengers known as prostaglandins. These are important for joint and muscle recovery, as well as numerous other important functions. Now we know that the omega-3 fats also activate genes that encourage fat burning and blunt fat storage. You need about 20–30% of your total daily calories to come from fat.

12 What's the right way to cheat on a diet?
It is actually beneficial for those eating a low-carb diet to cheat once a week by having a very high-carb day (at least 2g of carbs per pound of body weight). For those on a moderate-carb, maintenance diet, or trying to add muscle, try a cheat meal once per week—anything you want, like pizza or a burger and fries. And dessert. This one meal won't derail your progress, but will make a world of difference in your sanity while dieting. When you allow yourself this one cheat meal per week, it's a carrot you can dangle in front of yourself — you are actually less likely to cheat the rest of the week. After that cheat meal, most people feel satisfied and ready for another week of clean eating before cheating again.

13 Should I weigh my food before meals? What if I don't have a food scale?
You do not need to weigh all food. When you buy meat, the weight is on the package. You can estimate the weight of a chicken breast by dividing the number of chicken breasts in the package by the total weight of the package. For other foods, here's a helpful cheat sheet you can use in lieu of a food scale:

MEASURING STICK	FOOD
Ice-cream scoop	½ cup cooked rice/pasta/oatmeal
Tennis ball	1 medium fruit (apple/orange/pear)
Yo-yo	Bagel
Fist	4 oz chicken/beef/turkey/fish
Thumb	1 oz cheese
Handful	1 serving nuts (almonds/walnuts/cashews)

14 What are the best and worst condiments to use?
The worst condiments are those that contain high fructose corn syrup, as many ketchups and barbecue sauces do. Mustards are great, as the mustard seed has been shown to boost fat burning. And soy sauce is fine, too—in moderation—as it is low in calories.

15 Can I season my foods? Which seasonings are OK to use and which should I stay away from?
Yes, do yourself a favor and season your foods to enhance the flavor. It's easier to eat "clean" when the food tastes good. The absolute best seasonings and spices are cayenne pepper, garlic, and ginger, since these not only punch up the flavor of your foods, but also punch up your fat burning and also provide numerous other health benefits. Salt is fine, too, as you only need to worry about cutting sodium during the final week before a contest or photo shoot.

16 How will drinking alcohol affect my diet?
Alcohol is not as bad as you may think, as long as you keep in moderation. Research shows those who are moderate drinkers do not gain as much weight over the years as those who abstain. In fact, hard liquor and wine offer certain health benefits. Alcohol itself doesn't get converted into body fat; however, excessive alcohol can alter the biochemistry of the body to make fat storage easier. So try to keep it to a glass or two of alcohol once or twice per week.

17 Are some vegetables better than others?
All vegetables are good if you stick with true vegetables. True vegetables are low in starchy carbs, but high in fiber. These include foods like broccoli, asparagus, spinach, kale and cauliflower. Corn is high in starchy carbs, but it is technically not a veggie, even though most people think of it that way. Corn is actually a grain, much like wheat and rice. One cup of corn has over 40g of carbs, whereas one cup of chopped broccoli has only 6g. And, obviously, watch your intake of potatoes, which are classified as tubers. White potatoes are not only very starchy, but they digest very rapidly, which boosts insulin levels.

KNOW YOUR FATS

THE GOOD

> Monounsaturated fats lower total cholesterol and LDL cholesterol (the bad cholesterol) while increasing HDL cholesterol (the good cholesterol). Nuts (walnuts, almonds), avocados, and canola and olive oil are high in MUFAs. MUFAs have also been found to help in weight loss, particularly body fat.

> Polyunsaturated fats also lower total cholesterol and LDL cholesterol. Seafood like salmon and fish oil, as well as corn, soy, safflower, and sunflower oils are high in polyunsaturated fats. Omega-3 fatty acids belong to this group.

THE BAD

> Saturated fats raise total blood cholesterol as well as LDL cholesterol. Saturated fats are mainly found in animal products, such as meat, dairy, eggs and seafood. Some plant foods, such as coconut oil, palm oil, and palm kernel oil are also high in saturated fats.

> Trans fats were invented when scientists began to "hydrogenate" liquid oils for them to better withstand the food production process and give foods a longer shelf life. As a result of hydrogenation, trans fatty acids are formed. Trans fatty acids are found in many commercially packaged foods, in commercially fried food such as French fries from some fast-food chains, and in other packaged snacks such as microwave popcorn, as well as in vegetable shortening and hard-stick margarine.

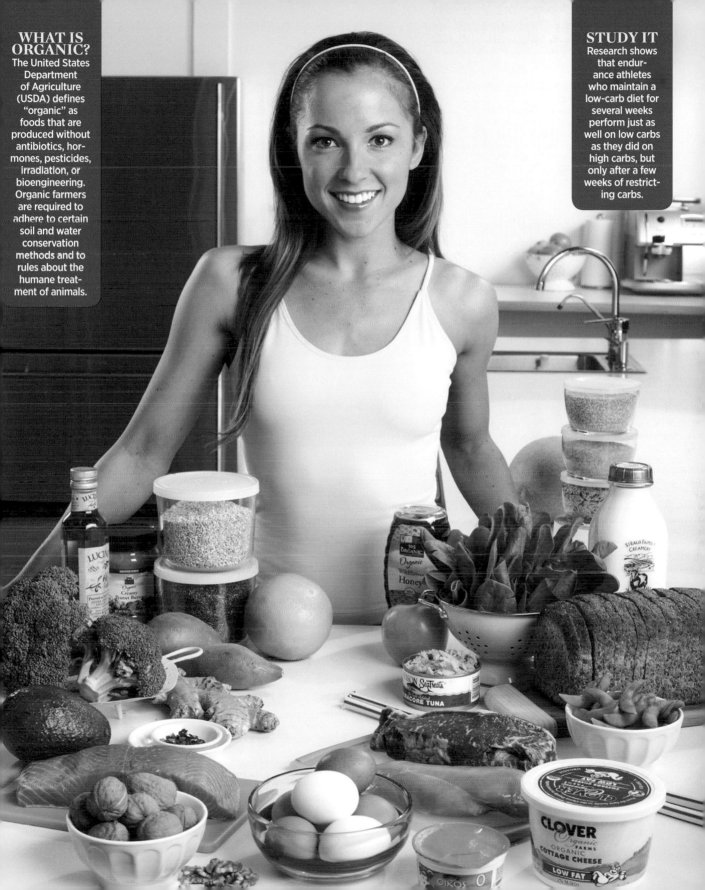

GOAL: Burn Fat One-Week Meal Plan

The following plan is designed for a woman weighing 140 pounds. When trying to lose weight during a rigorous exercise program, a good rule of thumb is to shoot for an intake of about 12 calories per pound of bodyweight. So for a 110-pound woman, total daily calories would be approximately 1,320; for a 150-pound woman, about 1,800.

A
TURKEY ROLLS
4 slices turkey deli meat
2 slices reduced-fat swiss cheese (Alpine Lace)
Place two slices of turkey together and lay one slice of cheese on top; spread mustard on cheese and roll into a tube and eat.

B
BREAKFAST BURRITO
1 large whole large egg
1 large egg white
1 slice reduced-fat American cheese
2 slices low-fat deli ham
1 10" whole-wheat pita
Heat tortilla in warm pan; fry ham in pan and place on tortilla; scramble eggs and cook in pan using nonstick cooking spray, add cheese and place on tortilla; roll tortilla into breakfast burrito.

C
CHILI CON CARNE
6 oz lean ground beef (90% lean)
¼ can (14½ oz) diced tomatoes with chilies
¼ medium onion (diced)
Brown beef in pan; add tomatoes and onion, ½ tsp ground cumin powder, 1 tsp chili pepper flakes, salt and pepper to taste.

D
OMELET
1 large whole egg
2 large egg whites
2 tbsp light cream cheese
½ cup raw spinach
Scramble the eggs in a pan with olive oil or nonfat cooking spray; flip eggs; mix together cream cheese and spinach in a bowl; spread cream cheese mixture onto cooked side of egg. Wait 30 seconds to ensure the other side of the egg is cooked, fold in half, wait 1 minute to melt cream cheese mixture.

E
BREAKFAST PIZZA

1 large whole egg
¼ cup fat-free mozzarella
¼ Boboli whole-wheat pizza crust
2 slices Jennie-O extra lean turkey bacon
Beat egg in bowl and slowly drizzle half over the crust; spread cheese over crust and drizzle the rest of the egg over the cheese; top with bacon; bake in oven at 450 degrees for about 10 minutes or until egg is cooked and cheese is melted.

MONDAY
BREAKFAST 1
1 scoop whey protein
½ large grapefruit
BREAKFAST 2
(30–60 minutes after B1)
Western Bagel Perfect 10 Healthy Grain Bagel
1 tbsp peanut butter
LATE-MORNING SNACK
2 large whole eggs (hard-boiled)
LUNCH
Turkey Rolls A Recipe
MIDDAY SNACK
3 oz albacore tuna (in water)
¼ cup low-fat cottage cheese
(Mix cottage cheese in tuna, add any desired vegetables.)
DINNER
6 oz shrimp
1 cup frozen stir-fry vegetables
¼ small ginger root, thinly sliced
1 tbsp soy sauce
(Stir-fry veggies and shrimp, then add soy sauce and ginger.)
2 cups mixed green salad (include spinach and raw broccoli)
1 tbsp olive oil and 1 tbsp balsamic vinegar (use as salad dressing)
NIGHTTIME SNACK
1 scoop casein protein
7 walnut halves
TOTALS: 1,565 CALORIES, 185G PROTEIN, 65G CARBS, 65G FAT

TUESDAY

BREAKFAST 1
1 scoop whey protein
½ large grapefruit
BREAKFAST 2
2 large whole eggs
3 slices Jennie-O extra-lean turkey bacon
1 cup cooked oatmeal
LATE-MORNING SNACK
½ cup cottage cheese
LUNCH
6 oz chicken breast
2 cups mixed green salad
1 tbsp olive oil and 1 tbsp balsamic vinegar (use as salad dressing)
MIDDAY SNACK
½ cup reduced-fat Greek yogurt
1 tbsp peanut butter
(Mix peanut butter in yogurt)
DINNER
6 oz salmon
½ cup mixed frozen veggies
2 cups mixed green salad (include spinach and raw broccoli)
1 tbsp olive oil and 1 tbsp balsamic vinegar (use as salad dressing)
NIGHTTIME SNACK
½ cup cottage cheese
2 tbsp salsa
(Mix salsa in cottage cheese.)
TOTALS: 1,715 CALORIES, 170G PROTEIN, 80G CARBS, 75G FAT

WEDNESDAY
BREAKFAST 1
1 scoop whey protein
½ large grapefruit
BREAKFAST 2
2 large whole eggs
1 whole egg white
⅛ cup fat-free cheddar cheese
(Make cheese omelet.)
1 whole-grain waffle (such as Van's)
2 tbsp fat-free Reddi-Wip
(Top waffle with whipped cream.)
Late-morning snack
1 scoop whey protein
1 tbsp peanut butter
LUNCH
3 oz albacore tuna (in water)
2 cups mixed green salad (include spinach and raw broccoli)

1 tbsp olive oil and 1 tbsp balsamic vinegar (use as salad dressing)
(Top salad with tuna.)
MIDDAY SNACK
2 slices low-fat American cheese
2 slices low-fat deli ham
¼ avocado
(Take one slice of ham and top with one slice of cheese. Place a slice of avocado in the middle and roll together. Repeat with the other slices of ham, cheese and avocado.)
DINNER
6 oz chicken breast
1 cup chopped broccoli
2 cups mixed green salad (include spinach and raw broccoli)
1 tbsp olive oil and 1 tbsp balsamic vinegar (use as salad dressing)
NIGHTTIME SNACK
1 scoop casein protein
TOTALS: 1,600 CALORIES, 180G PROTEIN, 65G CARBS, 65G FAT

THURSDAY
BREAKFAST 1
1 scoop whey protein
½ large grapefruit
BREAKFAST 2
Breakfast Burrito B Recipe
LATE-MORNING SNACK
1 oz fat-free cheese (Swiss, cheddar, Monterey jack)
2 slices turkey breast deli meat
(Slice cheese into two thin pieces and place in middle of turkey, roll up turkey and eat.)
7 walnut halves
LUNCH
3 oz albacore tuna (in water)
½ cup lowfat cottage cheese
(Mix tuna and cottage cheese together, add diced onions, carrots and peppers if desired.)
2 cups mixed green salad (include spinach and raw broccoli)
1 tbsp olive oil and 1 tbsp balsamic vinegar (use as salad dressing)
AFTERNOON SNACK
1 stick light mozzarella string cheese
DINNER
Taco Salad
4 oz lean ground turkey
¼ cup fat-free cheddar cheese
1 tbsp fat-free sour cream
4 tbsp salsa
1 cup shredded iceberg lettuce
½ medium tomato, diced
(Make taco salad: brown meat in frying pan

and add taco seasoning; place meat over bed of lettuce; add diced tomato, cheese, salsa and sour cream.)
NIGHTTIME SNACK
1 scoop casein protein
TOTALS: 1,500 CALORIES, 170G PROTEIN, 80G CARBS, 55G FAT

FRIDAY
BREAKFAST 1
1 scoop whey protein
½ large grapefruit
BREAKFAST 2
½ cup low-fat milk
½ cup Kashi Go Lean cereal
2 large whole eggs (scrambled, fried or hard boiled)
LATE-MORNING SNACK
¼ cup boiled soybeans (edamame)
1 stick light mozzarella string cheese
LUNCH
¾ cup low-fat cottage cheese
(Mix in any desired vegetables.)
MIDDAY SNACK
4 oz shrimp
1 tbsp seafood cocktail sauce
DINNER
Chili Con Carne C Recipe
2 cups mixed green salad (include spinach and raw broccoli)
1 tbsp olive oil and 1 tbsp balsamic vinegar (use as salad dressing)
NIGHTTIME SNACK
1 scoop casein protein
2 medium celery stalks
1 tbsp peanut butter
(Spread peanut butter into grooves of celery.)
TOTALS: 1,600 CALORIES, 170G PROTEIN, 75G CARBS, 65G FAT

SATURDAY
BREAKFAST 1
1 scoop whey protein
½ large grapefruit
BREAKFAST 2
Omelet D Recipe
½ whole-wheat English muffin
1 tbsp peanut butter
Late-morning snack
1 stick light mozzarella string cheese
2 medium celery stalks
1 tbsp peanut butter
(Spread peanut butter into grooves of celery.)
LUNCH
3 oz albacore tuna (in water)

1 tbsp light mayonnaise
3 whole-wheat crackers
(Add any desired vegetables to tuna salad and eat with crackers.)
MIDDAY SNACK
½ cup reduced fat Greek yogurt
7 walnut halves
(Mix walnuts in yogurt.)
DINNER
6 oz salmon
1 cup cooked cauliflower
2 cups mixed green salad
   (include spinach and raw broccoli)
1 tbsp olive oil and 1 tbsp balsamic vinegar (use as salad dressing)
NIGHTTIME SNACK
¾ cup low-fat cottage cheese
TOTALS: 1,635 CALORIES, 150G PROTEIN, 75G CARBS, 85G FAT

SUNDAY (HIGH-CARB "CHEAT" DAY)
BREAKFAST 1
1 scoop whey protein
1 large grapefruit
BREAKFAST 2
Breakfast Pizza E Recipe
4 oz (½ cup) orange juice
Late-morning snack
8 oz nonfat fruit yogurt
LUNCH
3 oz albacore tuna (in water)
1 tbsp fat-free mayonnaise
1 large (6.5") pita bread (white)
(Mix mayo in tuna to make tuna salad and add any veggies you desire. Scoop tuna salad into pita bread.)
1 cup sliced strawberries
4 tbsp fat-free Reddi-Wip
MIDDAY SNACK
1½ cups Kashi Go Lean cereal
1 cup low-fat Milk
DINNER
4 oz chicken breast
1 large sweet potato
2 tbsp fat-free sour cream
(Top potato with sour cream.)
2 cups mixed green salad (include spinach and raw broccoli)
1 tbsp olive oil and 1 tbsp balsamic vinegar (use as salad dressing)
NIGHTTIME SNACK
1 scoop casein protein
1 cup cooked oatmeal
TOTALS: 2,260 CALORIES, 190G PROTEIN, 300G CARBS, 40G FAT

TIME TO CHEAT Nutritional values for some of the more common cheat meals:	Quarter pounder with cheese and small fries (McDonalds) 740 calories 32g protein 37g fat 69g carbs 1,350mg sodium 9g sugar	Cheese Pizza, 1 slice (Domino's) 63 calories 4g protein 5g fat 1g carbs 208mg sodium 1g sugar	Double Hot Fudge Brownie Sundae (Ruby's) 1,108 calories 14g protein 47g fat 159g carbs 418mg sodium 125g sugar	Nachos Supreme (Taco Bell) 440 calories 12g protein 24g fat 42g carbs 680mg sodium 3g sugar	4 Chocolate chip cookies (Chips Ahoy) 190 calories 2g protein 9g fat 27g carbs 140mg sodium 13g sugar

GOAL: Build Lean Muscle One-Week Meal Plan

The following plan is designed for a woman weighing 140 pounds. When trying to gain lean muscle during a rigorous exercise program, a good rule of thumb is to shoot for an intake of about 13–15 calories per pound of bodyweight. So for a 110-pound woman, total daily calories would be between 1,430 to 1,650; for a 150-pound woman, about 1,950 to 2,250.

A
FRITTATA
2 large whole eggs
1 large egg white
¼ **cup** low-fat cottage cheese
½ **cup** chopped broccoli
½ medium onion (chopped)
In frying pan on medium heat, cook onions for about five minutes with fat-free cooking spray; add broccoli and cook for about five minutes; in a large bowl, mix eggs, and cottage cheese and add to pan, lift and rotate pan so that eggs are evenly distributed; as eggs set around the edges, lift to allow uncooked portions to flow underneath. Turn heat to low, cover the pan and cook until top is set. Invert onto a plate.

B
STIR-FRY
4 oz shrimp
1 large whole egg
½ **cup** cooked medium-grain brown rice
1 cup mixed frozen veggies
In a pan over medium heat cook shrimp in nonfat cooking spray, add boiled rice and vegetables, add scrambled egg and soy sauce if desired and cook for about 5–10 minutes, stirring frequently.

C
SPAGHETTI AND MEATBALLS
4 oz lean ground turkey
1 cup cooked spaghetti squash
¼ **cup** fat-free ricotta
Mix desired spices with ground turkey and roll into balls; add desired spices to sauce and cook meatballs in sauce until done. Cook spaghetti squash in a shallow baking pan with ½ inch of water in pan at 350 degrees in oven until tender. Scrape out spaghetti squash with fork to make spaghetti strings. Top spaghetti squash with meatballs and sauce, and spinach and top with ricotta.

D
BREAKFAST SANDWICH
1 large whole egg
1 slice reduced-fat American cheese
2 slices low-fat deli ham
1 whole-wheat English muffin
Make breakfast sandwich: toast muffin; fry ham in pan and place on one half of muffin; fry egg in pan using nonstick cooking spray and place on ham; top egg with cheese and cover with other muffin half to make breakfast sandwich.

MONDAY
BREAKFAST 1
1 scoop whey protein
½ small/medium cantaloupe
BREAKFAST 2
(30–60 minutes after B1)
2 large whole eggs
2 slices low-fat deli ham
¼ **cup** fat-free cheddar cheese
(Make ham-and-cheese omelet.)
1 cup cooked oatmeal
LATE-MORNING SNACK
4 oz reduced-fat Greek yogurt
½ **cup** blueberries
(Mix blueberries in yogurt.)
LUNCH
4 oz lean ground beef
1 whole-wheat hamburger bun
2 cups mixed green salad (include spinach)
1 tbsp olive oil and 1 tbsp balsamic vinegar (use as salad dressing)
MIDDAY SNACK
3 oz can chicken breast (such as Swanson)
1 tbsp light mayonnaise
5 whole-wheat crackers
(Mix mayo in chicken, eat on crackers.)
DINNER
6 oz chicken breast
1 cup chopped broccoli
2 cups mixed green salad (include spinach)
1 tbsp olive oil and 1 tbsp balsamic vinegar (use as salad dressing)

NIGHTTIME SNACK
¾ **cup** cottage cheese
2 tbsp salsa
(Mix salsa in cottage cheese.)
TOTALS: 1,835 CALORIES, 185G PROTEIN, 135G CARBS, 65G FAT

TUESDAY
BREAKFAST 1
1 scoop whey protein
1 large orange
BREAKFAST 2
2 large whole eggs
2 large egg whites
(Make scrambled eggs.)
1 whole-grain waffle (such as Van's)
1 tbsp maple syrup
LATE-MORNING SNACK
1 scoop whey protein
½ **cup** wheat germ
(Mix wheat germ in whey shake.)
LUNCH
4 oz turkey deli meat
1 tbsp light mayonnaise
2 slices Ezekiel 4:9 bread
(Make turkey sandwich.)
MIDDAY SNACK
½ **cup** low-fat cottage cheese
¼ **cup** sliced pineapple
(Mix pineapple in cottage cheese.)
DINNER
6 oz tilapia
1 cup broccoli
2 cups mixed green salad (include spinach)
1 tbsp olive oil and 1 tbsp balsamic vinegar (use as salad dressing)
NIGHTTIME SNACK
1 scoop casein protein
7 walnut halves
1 tbsp peanut butter
(Dip walnuts in peanut butter.)
TOTALS: 1,870 CALORIES, 190G PROTEIN, 145G CARBS, 60G FAT

WEDNESDAY
BREAKFAST 1
1 scoop whey protein
1 small apple
BREAKFAST 2
Frittata A Recipe
1 cup cooked oatmeal

LATE-MORNING SNACK
½ **cup** reduced-fat Greek yogurt
½ **cup** sliced strawberries
LUNCH
Stir-fry B Recipe
MIDDAY SNACK
½ **cup** low-fat cottage cheese
½ **cup** canned Mandarin oranges
DINNER
6 **oz** top sirloin steak
20 asparagus spears
2 **cups** mixed green salad (include spinach)
1 **tbsp** olive oil and 1 tbsp balsamic vinegar (use as salad dressing)
NIGHTTIME SNACK
1 **cup** reduced-fat Greek yogurt
1 **tsp** honey
2 **tbsp** roasted flaxseeds
(Mix honey and flaxseeds in yogurt.)
TOTALS: 1,900 CALORIES, 180G PROTEIN, 160G CARBS, 55G FAT

THURSDAY
BREAKFAST 1
1 scoop whey protein
½ medium cantaloupe
BREAKFAST 2
½ **cup** low-fat milk
½ **cup** Kashi Go Lean cereal
½ scoop whey protein
LATE-MORNING SNACK
2 **cups** mixed green salad (include spinach)
2 large whole eggs (hard-boiled and sliced)
¼ **cup** dry oatmeal
1 **tbsp** olive oil and 1 tbsp balsamic vinegar (use as salad dressing)
(Make salad by adding all ingredients together.)
LUNCH
5 **oz** packet seasoned tuna filets (such as StarKist)
½ **cup** cooked quinoa
1 **cup** mixed frozen veggies
MIDDAY SNACK
½ 10" whole-wheat pita (such as Mission Foods)
¼ **cup** reduced-fat cheddar cheese shredded
(Make cheese quesadilla: add cheese to one side of tortilla, fold in half and cook on medium heat in frying pan until cheese is melted.)
DINNER
6 **oz** salmon
2 **cups** mixed green salad (include spinach)

1 **tbsp** olive oil and 1 tbsp balsamic vinegar (use as salad dressing)
NIGHTTIME SNACK
¾ **cup** cottage cheese
2 **tbsp** salsa
TOTALS: 1,855 CALORIES, 165G PROTEIN, 130G CARBS 75G FAT

FRIDAY
BREAKFAST 1
1 scoop whey protein
1 small apple
BREAKFAST 2
¾ **cup** cottage cheese
½ **cup** Mandarin oranges (canned)
2 medium stalks celery
1 **tbsp** peanut butter
(Fill celery grooves with peanut butter.)
LATE-MORNING SNACK
1 scoop whey protein
½ **cup** wheat germ
(Mix whey and wheat germ together.)
LUNCH
4 **oz** turkey breast deli meat
1 **slice** reduced-fat American cheese
1 **tbsp** light mayonnaise
1 10" whole-wheat pita
MIDDAY SNACK
2 **oz** fat-free cheese
5 whole-wheat crackers
DINNER
6 **oz** tilapia
2 **cups** mixed green salad (include spinach)
1 **tbsp** olive oil and 1 tbsp balsamic vinegar (use as salad dressing)
NIGHTTIME SNACK
1 scoop casein protein
7 walnut halves
TOTALS: 1,915 CALORIES, 195G PROTEIN, 145G CARBS, 65G FAT

SATURDAY
BREAKFAST 1
1 scoop whey protein
1 large orange
BREAKFAST 2
2 large whole eggs
2 large egg whites
¼ **cup** reduced-fat cheddar cheese (shredded)
(Make cheese omelet.)
1 whole-wheat English muffin
1 **tbsp** peanut butter
(Spread peanut butter on toasted muffin.)

Late-morning snack
½ **cup** boiled soybeans
1 **cup** chicken noodle soup
LUNCH
3 **oz** albacore tuna (in water)
2 **cups** mixed green salad (include spinach)
1 **cup** beets (canned)
1 **oz** fat-free feta cheese
1 **tbsp** olive oil and 1 tbsp balsamic vinegar (use as salad dressing)
½ large whole-wheat pita bread, sliced into wedges
(Add ingredients to salad and eat with pita bread.)
MIDDAY SNACK
1 **cup** reduced-fat Greek yogurt
1 **tbsp** honey
DINNER
Spaghetti and Meatballs C
NIGHTTIME SNACK
¾ **cup** cottage cheese
TOTALS: 2,000 CALORIES, 180G PROTEIN, 170G CARBS, 70G FAT

SUNDAY (HIGH CARB "CHEAT" DAY)
BREAKFAST 1
1 scoop whey protein
½ medium cantaloupe
BREAKFAST 2
Breakfast Sandwich D
LATE-MORNING SNACK
½ **cup** reduced-fat Greek yogurt
½ **cup** blueberries
LUNCH
4 **oz** turkey deli meat
2 **slices** Ezekiel 4:9 bread
2 **cups** mixed green salad (include spinach)
1 **tbsp** olive oil and 1 tbsp balsamic vinegar (use as salad dressing)
MIDDAY SNACK
½ 10" whole-wheat pita (Mission Foods)
¼ **cup** fat-free cheddar
(Make cheese quesadilla.)
DINNER (CHEAT MEAL)
3 **slices** pepperoni pizza
12-oz Budweiser
1 **cup** ice cream
NIGHTTIME SNACK
½ **cup** low-fat cottage cheese
2 **tbsp** salsa
TOTALS: 2,500 CALORIES, 160G PROTEIN, 255G CARBS, 75G FAT

ALCOHOL CHOICES

Red wine *(5-oz serving):*
125 calories, 0g protein, 4g carbs, 0g fat (108 calories come from alcohol content).
Low in calories due to low sugar content; contains resveratrol, a super anti-oxidant that may combat cancer and reduce signs of aging (among other benefits).

White wine *(5-oz serving):*
121 calories, 0g protein, 4g carbs, 0g fat (105 calories come from alcohol content).
Low in calories and carbs, but has less phenols and antioxidants than red wine. White wine is better than many alcohols, but red wine wins on all counts.

Beer *(10-oz serving):*
126 calories, 2g protein, 10g carbs, 0g fat (76 calories come from alcohol content)
Good for an antioxidant boost, but with a lot of calories on the side. Light beers come closer to the carb content of white wine, and are the healthier choice.

Margarita *(5-oz serving):*
230 calories, 0.5g protein, 10g carbs, 0g fat (189 calories come from alcohol content).
A margarita is made with tequila, triple sec, lime juice, sugar and ice and is usually served on the rocks. Not typically considered nutritious, the alcohol and sugar provide the calorie count and the lime juice proffers some vitamin C. Traditionally served in a salt-rimmed glass, the margarita is also high in sodium.

Mojito *(5-oz serving):*
215 calories, 0g protein, 8.5g carbs, 0g fat (179 calories come from alcohol content).
Because the flavor, for the most part, comes from fresh mint and limes (and a teaspoon or two of sugar), the calorie count here is lighter than a cocktail mixed with flavored syrup.

The 15 Best Fat-Burning Foods

1) Walnuts
All nuts do contain some amount of the omega-3 fat alpha-linolenic acid, but most only contain trace amounts. The real fat hero in most nuts is monounsaturated fats. Walnuts are actually a rich source of omega-3s. One ounce provides almost 3g of alpha-linolenic acid.

2) Ginger
Used for centuries to help relieve digestive upset/disturbances, ginger can also help reduce inflammation, boost blood flow to muscles, and aid muscle recovery. It has also has been shown to boost calorie burn when eaten.

3) Oatmeal
This very slow-digesting carb keeps blood sugar and insulin levels low, so fat burning can stay high. In fact, research has shown that athletes who consume slow-digesting carbs in the morning burn more fat throughout the entire day and during workouts than those consuming fast-digesting carbs.

4) Avocado
The monounsaturated fats found in avocados are burned readily for fuel during exercise and actually encourage fat burning. Avocados also contain a very interesting carb called manno-heptulose, a sugar that actually blunts insulin release and enhances calcium absorption, both of which are critical for encouraging fat loss.

5) Salmon
This fish is one of the richest sources of the omega-3 essential fats EPA and DHA. Unlike flaxseeds, which provide a type of omega-3 that has to be converted into EPA and DHA, salmon provides your body a direct supply of them with no conversion required. This way you know you're getting a direct supply of the fats that turn on fat burning and block fat storage.

6) Soybeans (edamame)
Soybeans are the direct origin of soy protein, which has been shown to build muscle as efficiently as other forms of protein like whey and beef. Soy has also been shown to aid fat loss, possibly by decreasing appetite and calorie intake.

7) Water
This just may be your best ally in fighting body-fat. Studies have shown that drinking 2 cups of cold water can boost metabolic rate by 30%. It has been estimated that drinking about 2 cups of cold water before breakfast, lunch, and dinner every day for a year can burn 17,400 extra calories, which translates into a little more than 5 pounds of body fat!

8) Flaxseeds
They contain the essential omega-3 fatty acid alpha linolenic acid. These omega-3 fats have been found to turn on genes that stimulate fat burning and turn off genes that increase fat storage.

9) Grapefruit
A study from the Scripps Clinic (San Diego, California) reported that subjects eating half of a grapefruit or drinking 8 oz of grapefruit juice three times a day while maintaining their normal diet lost an average of 4 pounds over 12 weeks—and some lost more than 10 pounds without even dieting! Results were likely due to grapefruit's ability to reduce insulin levels and to a chemical in grapefruit known as naringin, which prevents fat from being stored in the body.

10) Honey
Yes, it's a sugar, but it's fairly low on the glycemic index. Keeping insulin levels low and steady is critical for maintaining a fat-burning environment in your body. Honey is also a rich source of nitric oxide (NO) metabolites; ultimately, that means it actually encourages fat release from the body's fat cells.

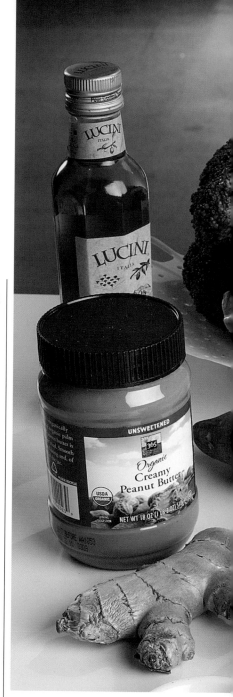

11) Peanut butter
Another source of helpful monounsaturated fat that can actually aid fat loss. What's funny is that many food manufacturers make low-fat peanut butters! Of course, they replace these healthy monounsaturated fats with carbs, namely sugar. Avoid these and stick with natural peanut butters that don't add the type of fat you surely want to avoid—trans fats.

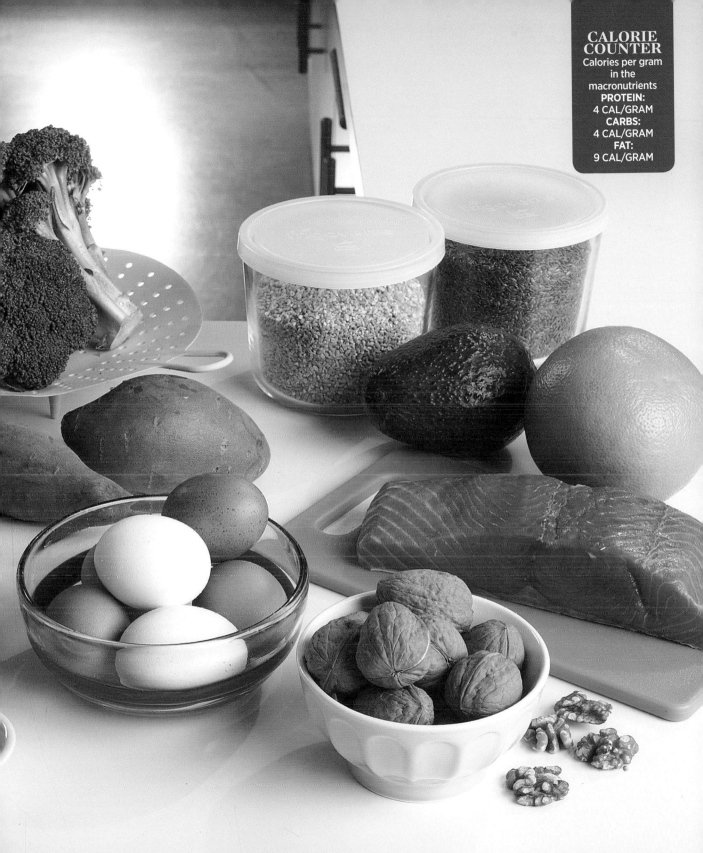

CALORIE COUNTER
Calories per gram in the macronutrients
PROTEIN:
4 CAL/GRAM
CARBS:
4 CAL/GRAM
FAT:
9 CAL/GRAM

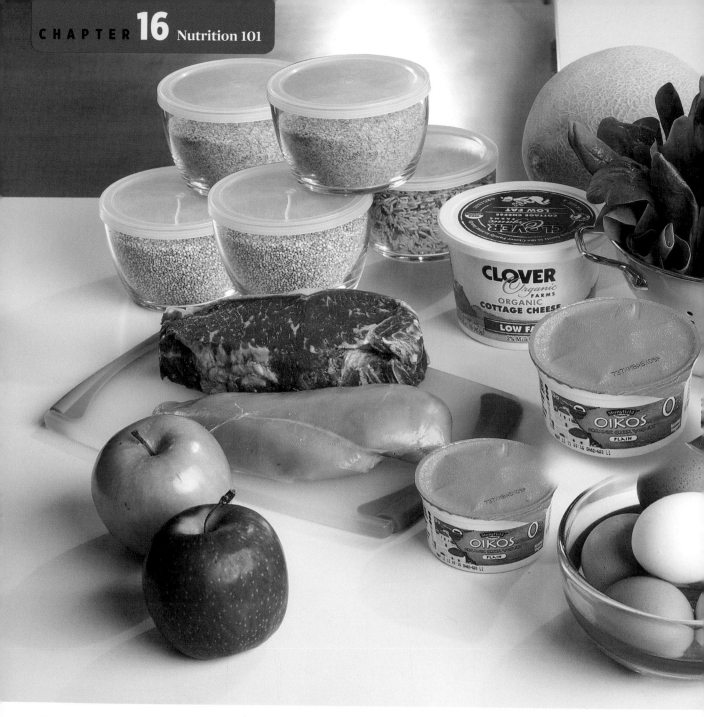

12) Eggs

Yes, we listed eggs in the muscle-building foods section later in this chapter. So how can it also be a fat-burning food? Research supports the notion that those who start their day with eggs not only eat fewer calories throughout the day, but also lose significantly more body fat.

13) Chili pepper flakes

Hot peppers contain the active ingredient capsaicin, a chemical that can enhance calorie burning at rest as well as reduce hunger and food intake. The boost in calorie burn is particularly enhanced when capsaicin is used with caffeine.

14) Broccoli

This fibrous carb doesn't provide many net carbs or calories, but it can make you feel full—one reason why it's a great food for getting lean. Broccoli also contains phytochemicals that can help enhance fat loss.

The 15 Best Lean-Muscle Building Foods

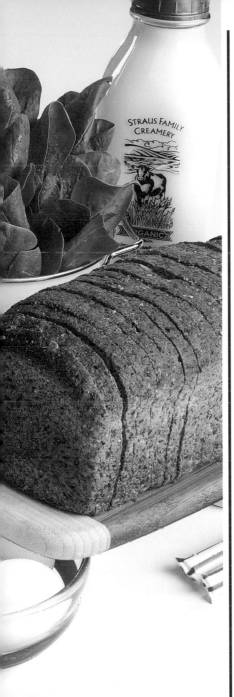

1) Beef (from grass-fed cattle)

Beef is important for building lean muscle due to its protein content, cholesterol, zinc, B vitamins, and iron content. Beef from grass-fed cattle have much higher levels of conjugated linoleic acid (CLA) than conventionally raised cattle, which gives you a boost in shedding bodyfat and building lean muscle.

2) Beets

A good source of betaine, also known as tri-methylglycine, this nutrient not only enhances liver and joint repair, but also has been shown in clinical research to increase muscle strength and power. Beets also provide an NO boost which can ehance energy and aid recovery.

3) Brown rice

A slow-digesting whole grain that provides you longer-lasting energy throughout the day, and during workouts. Brown rice also can help boost your growth hormone (GH) levels, which are critical for encouraging lean muscle growth, fat loss, and strength gains.

4) Oranges

Another good fruit that can actually help to boost muscle growth, strength, and endurance, especially when eaten before workouts.

5) Cantaloupe

Due to it's relatively low fructose content, this melon is one of the few fruits that is actually a fast-digesting carb. That makes it a good carb to have first thing in the morning after a long night of fasting and one of the few good fruits to eat after workouts.

6) Cottage cheese (organic)

Rich in casein protein, cottage cheese is a great go-to protein source, especially before bed. Casein protein is the slowest-digesting protein you can eat, meaning it prevents your muscles from being used as an energy source while you fast during the night.

7) Eggs

Eggs are known as the perfect protein, but their ability to boost lean muscle and strength gains isn't due to just the protein alone. It gets a lot of help from the yolks, where the cholesterol is found. If you're worried about your cholesterol shooting up from eating the yolks, cholesterol from eggs has been shown to decrease the amount of LDL (bad) cholesterol particles associated with atherosclerosis.

8) Milk (organic)

Contains both whey and casein and is rich in the amino acid glutamine. Organic milk has about 70% more omega-3 fatty acids than conventional milk.

9) Quinoa

A complete protein in addition to being a slow digesting carb, quinoa has been linked with an increase in insulinlike growth factor-1 (IGF-1) levels, an important factor associated with lean muscle and strength gains.

10) Wonka Pixy Stix

These contain dextrose, meaning this carb doesn't even need to be digested—it literally goes straight into your bloodstream, getting those carbs straight to your muscles for the fastest recovery possible after workouts.

11) Spinach

A good source of glutamine, the amino acid that is important for lean muscle growth. In addition to glutamine, spinach can increase muscle strength and endurance.

12) Apples

The specific polyphenols in apples help to increase muscle strength and prevent muscle fatigue, allowing you to train harder for longer. Other research also shows that these polyphe-

15) Olive oil

Like avocados, olive oil is a great source of monounsaturated fats. Not only do they lower levels of the "bad" type of cholesterol and improve cardiovascular health, but they're also more likely to be burned as fuel, which means they're less likely to be sticking around your midsection.

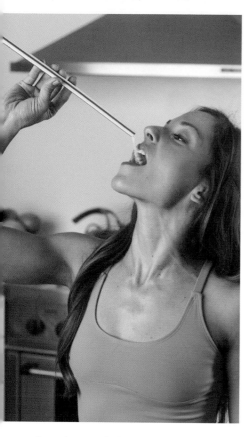

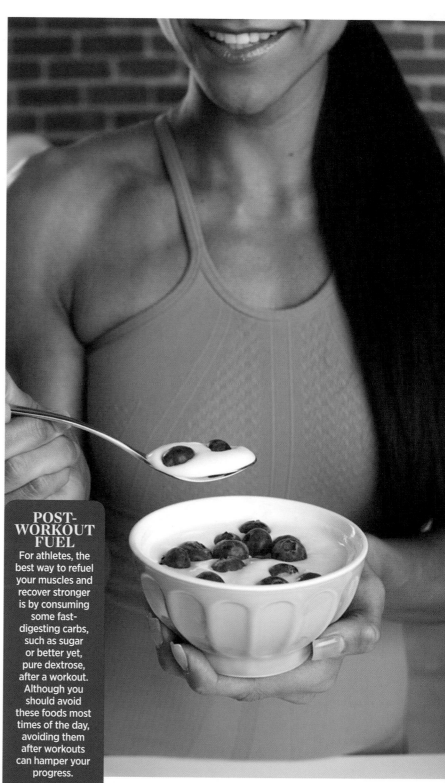

nols can increase fat burning as well. That's why it's a good idea to make apples a pre-workout carb source.

13) Greek yogurt

Like plain yogurt, Greek yogurt starts from the same source: milk. Greek yogurt, however, has more protein (a whopping 20g per cup) and fewer carbs (9g per cup) than regular yogurt (16g protein, 16g carbs per cup). It's also a good source of casein protein.

14) Ezekiel 4:9 Bread

Ezekiel bread is made from organic sprouted whole grains. Because it contains grains and legumes, the bread is a complete protein, which means it contains all nine of the amino acids your body can't produce on its own—the ones needed for lean muscle growth.

15) Wheat germ

Rich in zinc, iron, selenium, potassium, and B vitamins, high in fiber and protein, with a good amount of branched-chain amino acids (BCAAs), arginine, and glutamine. This makes wheat germ a great source of slow-digesting carbohydrates and a quality protein that's a perfect food before workouts.

POST-WORKOUT FUEL

For athletes, the best way to refuel your muscles and recover stronger is by consuming some fast-digesting carbs, such as sugar or better yet, pure dextrose, after a workout. Although you should avoid these foods most times of the day, avoiding them after workouts can hamper your progress.